The Cure
For All Disease

BY
TERRY COOKSEY

COVER ART
BY
TERRY COOKSEY

All questions about this book, whether it be about obtaining quantity discounts for books, requests to sell or distribute books or questions about content in books must be sent to:
inquiries@americanpublishing.us

ISBN-13: 978-1-499719-36-9
ISBN-10:   1-499719-36-1
Copyright © 2014 American Publishing US

Library of Congress Control Number: 2014933223

The Cure For All Disease

The Cure For All Disease

Table of Contents

ISBN-13: 978-1-499719-36-9
ISBN-10:   1-499719-36-1
Copyright © 2014 American Publishing US

Library of Congress Control Number: 2014933223

PREFACE

The Cure For All Disease is the Owner's Manual for your body.

I know that the title states something that few can accept as being true at this time. But the fact is, that there is a cure for all disease. And that is what you are about to discover. The results you get by doing what I say to cure you of all disease, is what is important.

There are 150,000,000 Americans who are permanently sick with one or more chronic diseases. The rest of the country is sick most of the time. No one calls this most devastating plague in the planet's history "a plague". But what else can you have when doctors refuse to cure anyone, in order to stuff their bank accounts with all the cash they can squeeze out of you.

Real doctors cure you. And up until drug corporations started patenting their chemical drugs in 1939, about 85% of Americans relied on Healers when it came to their health and well-being.

And what we have to do is return that way of curing almost everyone. But we also have to avoid the saturation of poisons in your food, drinks, water and personal hygiene items.

You also have to give your body the nutrients it needs to stay healthy and function properly. That requires taking vitamin supplements to get enough Vitamin C, Magnesium and Omega-3.

Any person who is sick needs to take measures to reverse the acidity of their body. Doing so causes disease to slowly fade away. I will tell you how you can reverse the acidic state of your body, and do so for pennies a day.

I will tell you some quick cures to some major diseases. Among those are migraines, kidney stones, heart arrhythmia, gout and more.

You can make major improvements in your health by taking Magnesium. When you find out all the things your body needs Magnesium for, you will begin to understand why your body is in poor health. Without Magnesium, over 300 body metabolisms do not occur or occur very little. As you continue without enough Magnesium for longer and longer periods of time, your body continues without the metabolisms that require ample Magnesium to happen.

The same is true about the acidity of your body. The more acidic, the more body metabolisms cease to occur. And as you continue to bombard your body with more and more poisons, those poisons begin to accumulate in places in your body. These accumulations of poisons in parts of your body is what is called disease.

This book goes after the cause of all disease. And without those poisons entering your body, disease will stay out of your body.

POISONS CAUSE ALL DISEASES.

And even the 20% of diseases that are said to be caused by germs and viruses, could not exist without your body being acidic from saturating it with more poisons than your body can remove.

I made this book short to make it easy for anyone to cure themselves of all their diseases. This includes headaches and heartburn. Both of them are common diseases that rare few even call "disease". But the same things that cure cancer, kidney disease and heart disease, also cure you of the lesser diseases such as headaches and heartburn.

Cure means to restore to health. And that is what this book teaches you to do. You can cure yourself of every disease you have WHILE you still listen to your doctors; except the part about death and there's no cure!

Everything I tell you to do is Natural and costs very little. You can expect to invest up to $150 for water filters. Then spend $20-$30 a month on the vitamins and a couple other things, to get you cured. So, in one year you will have spent a maximum of $510 to cure yourself of every disease you have.

I have written four other books on cures. They all tell you the same cure for all disease that is in this book. So I wrote this book to make the transition from talking about diseases, to talking about how to restore your body to health to rid it of all disease.

See, it's not really important what diseases you have. What's important is restoring your body to health.

This should be taught to children early in their lives. But as long as money continues to be far more important to doctors than human lives, the only chance you have to escape disease and an early death, is to use the science in this book to cure yourself.

For those who can choose Life over Death and well-being over permanent disease, let's get started on the best thing that could ever happen to anyone with chronic disease.

My Final Words at the end of the book is to talk to you about the things you need to know to make sure you don't get fooled by doctors and their complete refusal to cure anyone. Everything else is the information your body needs to heal itself.

Read on and see for yourself.............

1 - Introduction

After writing four books on cures, I have learned a whole lot of things I didn't know at those times. I didn't know that I had discovered the cure for all disease when I wrote my first book. But what I really did was discover laws of physics that dictate the health of our human bodies.

The most overwhelming mistake that everyone makes is going to doctors for cures. Doctors have no cures. So it is clearly insane to go to a doctor if you want to be cured. But this insanity goes deeper. Not only does everyone go to doctors for cures they never get, they never look elsewhere for any cures. And until you snap out of this robotic hypnotic trance, you will remain without cures for any of your diseases.

I became the first person to cure myself of chronic kidney disease in the past 75 years. Before the first patented drug in 1939, we actually cured ourselves of most every disease. But now with 150,000,000 Americans who are permanently sick, doctors feel no need to cure anyone. Even if doctors wanted to cure anyone, how could they; since doctors aren't taught cures in any of the medical schools.

So even when I went to the doctors to cure me of what turned out to be kidney disease, I not only didn't get cured by doctors, there was never any chance of me being cured by going to doctors.

I want to make it very clear at the very beginning of this book that I am not going to teach you how to avoid doctors. What I AM teaching you is how to cure yourself of all diseases. And as long as you think doctors are going to cure you, there is no chance you will ever be cured.

When you get past that mental block, you begin learning the Laws of Physics to cure yourself. Don't let the term "the Laws of Physics" make you think this is something only a few can understand. You know that water is always wet. That is one Law of Physics.

Throughout this book you will learn how to use Laws of Physics to cure your body of any and all diseases. A real simple example of using a Law of Physics to cure yourself is by using a highly alkaline natural substance to neutralize the excess acid we all call heartburn, aka acid reflux. Mix ½ teaspoon baking soda in 4-6 ounces of filtered water and drink when you have heartburn. You use this same thing to cure gout.

Gout is Uric acid crystals. Again, by using a highly alkaline natural substance like baking soda, we neutralize those Uric acid crystals known as gout. We use filtered water because it doesn't have the chlorine, fluoride and other poisons in it as unfiltered tap water does. This becomes very important once you realize that all disease requires an acidic body to exist in.

What I am teaching you to do is to RESTORE YOUR ENTIRE BODY TO HEALTH which will rid your body of all diseases. Up until this point in my life, I have called it cures. And with that comes all this talk about this disease, that disease, my disease and so on. Once a doctor defines the problem with your body they tell you the name of that isolated part of your body that isn't functioning properly. But no matter what disease or diseases doctors tell you that you have, the fact is that you have a whole body problem.

Your body produces cancer cells daily. But once your body is acidic, those same poisons that made your body acidic are now causing organs or other parts of your body to stop functioning normally. This is what doctors call disease. But the only reason doctors call it "chronic" disease is because they REFUSE to cure anyone in order to maximize their income off treating your diseases, instead of curing them as all real Physicians do. We have plenty of doctors but no Physicians, Healers.

The Laws of Physics can not be patented. Nature can't be patented. So doctors ignore all cures, since all cures are natural. Your body is natural. But nothing doctors do is natural! The very idea of pretending to help your natural body without using anything natural is the most perverted quackery that could ever be concocted by anyone!

The most common questions people around the world ask me, are about whether natural things will hurt them! My answers are redundant and shout how bizarre it is for anyone to even think natural things could hurt you. But this is the mentality that doctors create. Doctors' prescription drugs and other UN-natural ways kill over 100,000 people each year in the US alone. But to this day, no one has died from taking natural things like vitamins, herbs or even the most opposed natural medicine of all, marijuana.

But marijuana is illegal and the deadly drugs made by corporations and prescribed by doctors are not! Such contempt for human life can never be tolerated by civilized people! Do something about the 100's of thousands of people being killed by these deadly drugs. And stop using the Police and Federal government to insure this mass slaughter and imprisoning people for using what use to be the #1 medicine in the USA. This is what has forced everyone to either take the deadly chemical drugs that only harm our bodies further OR endure endless pain and suffering and an early death.

Doctors and the medical profession have been coming out with one claim after another telling the Public that everything natural will harm and kill us. It's quite bizarre, due to the fact that doctors claim they can't advise anyone about the use of vitamins and herbs. I believe that is the law, rules, for them. I asked my first nephrologist about using specific herbal cleanses and his reply was "I couldn't tell you that. I've never studied herbs before."

Now that statement seems OK at first until you remember the synonym for herb is "medicine"!!! Any plant that has been used as a medicine is classified as an herb. But yet, doctors don't use herbs, natural medicines. ALL their "medicines" are synthetic man-made chemicals. And although many of their chemical "medicines" help you temporarily, fact is that your body works to remove 100% of all those drugs you take. But natural things have the ability to remain in your body and become part of your body.

One example of that would be how every cell in your body contains Calcium. So you have to give your body the Calcium it needs to do everything it can do for your body. Your body has to have enough Magnesium to dissolve the Calcium in order for Calcium to be used by your body. And when you don't have enough Magnesium, over 300 body metabolisms no longer occur. This causes kidney and bladder stones and bone spurs, irregular heart beats, high blood pressure, bone spurs, a weakened immune system and a host of other break downs in your body.

These sciences are just part of what you will learn from this book. What you will really do is discover the sciences that made you sick in the first place, and the sciences that restore your body to health and cure you of any and all diseases. What doctors call disease, with all of its many names, is what I see as something wrong with your entire body.

When you have cancer, it's because your body couldn't remove all the poisons going in your body AND keep removing cancer cells fast enough to keep a cluster of cancer cells from accumulating in places in your body. If you had not abused your own body with all those sugars, white flour, animal products and chlorinated water, it would never have even been scientifically possible for cancer or any disease to exist in your body!

I will give you the basic cure for all diseases to begin what you must do to rid your body of all diseases. You have to remember that poisons equal diseases. Since poisons cause all disease, getting rid of the CAUSE of all disease is the way to cure and prevent all disease. But the biggest problem you have when trying to reduce the amount of poisons that enter your body, is that our entire food, drinks and water supplies are saturated with deadly poisons. And corporations use lots of deceit to trick you into believing their toxic products are not only safe, but good and healthy.

I will tell about that deceit and how to see through it. But what I am going to do, is make this as short and simple as I can in the next chapter. Then I will tell you other things you can do to improve the health of your body and speed your healing. I won't be focusing on changing your attitude, so you can be cured, until My Final Words.

I did that in all my other books on cures because all you hear from doctors and the medical profession is that there is no cure for any disease. So I spent the majority of those books trying to get people to accept the fact that there have always been cures for all diseases. Before the first chemical drugs were patented, starting in 1939, doctors cured every disease there is. The end of good doctors pretty much ended with Jonas Salk, who created the polio vaccine and gave it to mankind as a gift; not for money.

So cures have faded away and been replaced by the endless medical treatments, tests and procedures they can make money off of. And that is a huge tidal wave of deceit to get through, just so you will even consider you COULD be cured. All you hear is "There's no cure". But we had cures for every disease up until 1939. And we found cures for diseases as they were needed. But not after Jonas Salk's polio vaccine!

The information in this book needs to be done in order to bring the results it is intended to bring. So you don't have to waste your time judging what is stated in this book. All you have to do is DO what is stated and you get the results stated in this book. These sciences occur inside your bodies. So that is where these sciences bring the stated results.

I can't take any credit for these scientific Laws of Physics. They exist for you and everyone to discover and use to change the health of your bodies for the better, and restore your natural body to health to rid it of all disease.

I have been sharing these medical sciences with people all around the world who are getting better. Some cured themselves of a variety of diseases doing what I shared in my books and on my Facebook pages for my books.

Although Facebook is intolerable to many people because of all the drama and offensive political and religious hate speech, I have been able to help a lot of people in the Philippines, Nigeria, South Africa, Lebanon, Turkey, the UK, Australia, New Zealand and many more countries through the Facebook pages for my books How to Avoid Dialysis and Cure Kidney Disease, The Cure For Cancer and Natural Healing BOOK of CURES.

If you wish to contact me personally, just go to any of those pages and send me a private message or ask a question on any of the posts. Although all the information you need is in my books and posted on those Facebook pages, there are still questions you may have.

There is a cure for all disease. And that cure is all natural and costs you very little. The cost to restore your body back to health will be about $75 to $150 up front for water and shower filters, and $10 to $30 monthly for vitamins, baking soda and such. All you gotta do is decide if your life is worth that investment, then get science working FOR you to cure you and restore your entire body back to a healthy state.

So for all of you who care about your own health and lives, let's get to the information that will restore your body to health and rid you of every disease you have. The chances of you curing yourself with these sciences is the same as the chances of water being wet – which is 100% of the time.

2 - Time for Your Healing to Begin

What it takes to cure you of any and all disease is so simple and costs so very little that it is very hard for most people to understand how it could cure you. But getting rid of your diseases is not the focus of what I am telling you. You have to accept the fact that you have not been taking care of your body, even though you aren't eating any differently than the vast majority do.

But the food supplies have become so depleted of any real nutritional value that there is no chance of our food supplies nourishing your body properly. I mean there is no chance of getting the nutrients your body must have to function properly. So unless you are a vegetarian who eats lots of fresh raw produce, then your failure to take vitamin supplements assures that you will develop serious diseases; which are termed as chronic since doctors REFUSE to cure anyone.

Disease is what doctors give all these names to for all the different ways the effects of habitual mass poisoning show up in your body. If cancer cells are not removed by pure water and anti-oxidants faster than your body produces cancer cells, they amass in places in your body. If they accumulate in your liver, doctors call it "liver cancer". If those same cancer cells amass in your brain, doctors call it "brain cancer".

So you have doctors giving you their specific treatments for each of these cancers they gave different names to; although the cure for every cancer is the same. And the cure for all disease is basically the same. But there are things you can do that will restore your liver, pancreas, stomach, colon and other parts of your body faster, as long as you are following the basic cure for all diseases. A good example of this would be diabetes.

You can take Taurine, Cinnamon and digestive enzymes to speed the healing of your pancreas. Taurine is a powerful anti-oxidant, detox, you can take for your pancreas. Cinnamon helps control glucose very well. And the digestive enzymes relieve your pancreas of having to produce large amounts of enzymes to get the chunks of food digested that you didn't chew up well.

Here is the summary of what you have to do to restore your body to health and rid your body of all diseases:

- clean your water up with filters and drink plenty
- correct your major diet deficiencies
- reverse the acidic state of your body that allows disease
- clean up your diet including what you drink
- Look for every source of chemicals you put in your body or comes in contact with your body or the air you breathe; and avoid any further use or contact with those sources of chemicals

The first 3 things are pretty easy to get done. But the other 2 things listed are where all the complications are. This is because of all the massive deceit in advertisements, product labels, an offensively corrupt FDA and how it has become normal for us to deceive ourselves about poisons in our food, drinks, water and personal hygiene items.

In my other books on cures there are 3 chapters called "Poisons In Your" Food, Drinks and Water. I take 3 chapters to tell you how to recognize and avoid the saturation of poisons in our food, drinks and water. But in this book I am determined to make it much easier for you to rid your body of all disease and understand the natural sciences that dictate your body's health. In my first 4 books on cures, I explained how I cured myself of chronic kidney disease; and in the process, cured myself of all 11 diseases I had.

But since then, I realized what I did was restore my body to health. For me to do that I had to focus on what I was drinking, because I had the best food diet of anyone I knew. No one told me "WATCH WHAT YOU DRINK". And being blind to that, I drank my way all the way to kidney failure, heart disease, gout, arthritis, daily heartburn and headaches, bleeding gums and intestines, and teeth falling out of my mushy rotten gums for 7 or 8 years!

The sciences I used to restore my body to health and end all 10 diseases I had, AND the bladder stones I cured myself of in 1996, are what I am about to share with you. And as a result of what effects these sciences do for all of you who put them to use, I will now tell you what you need to restore your body to a healthy state. These are the things you should have been doing all of your life! But because of all the illegal mass poisoning of the entire population of the Earth by corporations, we have slowly been deceived and seduced into believing all these poisons are safe and do our bodies no harm.

But poisons have never been safe. And they're not safe just because they're in your food, drinks and water, Or because the FDA certifies all these toxic chemicals as "safe"... Or whatever excuse you have for NOT accepting the fact that POISONS ARE NOT SAFE or have no consequences. The result of these poisons are every disease that exists! Deal with the CAUSE of all disease to get rid of all disease. And POISONS CAUSE ALL DISEASE.

Pure Water – The Very Essence of Life

I believe the quality of your health is equal to the quality of your water. Every living thing requires water in order to exist and survive. That is real evident when it comes to restoring and maintaining the health of your body.

But even though Nature's water is the very essence of Life itself, almost all the water we have comes with chlorine and fluoride already in it. This makes your water the main source of poisons going into your body. That includes your drinking water and your shower water. And for that reason, and the fact that your body is 80% water, let me start off by telling you how to give yourself safe natural water.

So how do you provide you and your family with safe, natural water, free of the disease causing poisons that saturate our water supplies?

Just get a shower filter, a multi-stage fluoride filter and avoid all bottle water. Easy enough, right? Well, it sounds easy. But finding these filters is not so easy. In the City of 70,000 I live in, you couldn't buy a shower filter at any store in this area until 2013. I still can't even buy a fluoride water filter. I had to buy them online. So I am going to tell you where to buy them online.

Get a multi-stage fluoride filter to filter out 99% of the chlorine, most fluoride and every impurity in your tap water. The link for the filter we buy is: http://www.purewateressentials.com/ct-00145.html

For a shower filter, go to Ebay and SEARCH for CRYSTAL QUEST 3 Stage KDF Carbon SHOWER Water Filter. This will give you an assortment of shower filters and replacement filters. A shower filter is just a tubular shaped cylinder about 4-5 inches long that screws on your shower between the water pipe and the shower head.

Chlorine destroys the oxygen in every cell it comes in contact with. That includes the cells inside your body, your hair, scalp and skin, and your lungs. Every bit of chlorinated water you drink destroys oxygen in every cell it comes in contact with. Chlorine kills your gut flora, bacteria, until your body can remove it. This weakens your immune system at least as bad as anti-biotics do. Same thing when you use chlorinated water for cooking.

But in the shower you are doing the greatest harm to your skin, lungs and immune system. That chlorinated fluoridated water is soaking every pore on your body. The more that soaking continues, the wider your pores expand. That increases the amount of chlorine and fluoride that enters your body through your pores. Add to that, the amount of steam you are breathing in the shower, and you are doing enough to give yourself most any disease(s).

The benefits of a shower filter also ends your dandruff and those red itchy spots you have after a shower; as well as ending your dry hair problem too. If you take baths, run your bath water into the tub through a shower filter.

The best benefit a water filter for your drinking water brings you is the end of all that chlorine killing the good bacteria in your digestive system. As chlorine slowly kills most of the good bacteria, your barren stomach makes you feel like you are hungry most of the time; even an hour after eating.

Until you get those water filters, it's your liver and kidneys that are going to have to filter out all that chlorine, fluoride and other poisons and debris in your water supply. Your body will sustain all that damage from all that chlorine and fluoride that entered your body. And all you have to do is get a shower filter and a water filter and let those filters remove all that chlorine, debris and fluoride, so that it never enters your body through your mouth, lungs and pores. This relieves your kidneys and liver from having to remove these large amounts of chlorine and fluoride.

These filters will cost you about $150 up front. $25 every 12-18 months to replace your shower filter cartridge. And another $110 every 10 years to replace your counter-top fluoride filter I gave you the link for. That would be a cost of $275 every ten years. And don't forget what that $27 a year does for you. That is the reason you make this small investment. Compare that to the cost of a kidney transplant at over $262,000 and water filters are a super bargain! And kidney transplants are the least expensive; with Heart and Intestine transplant first year costs running $1,000,000 and more.

Once you have your filters installed, it's time for you to start drinking water daily at the rate of about 1-ounce for every 2 pounds of body weight. There is nothing that will clean out, detox, your entire body like a constant supply of pure water does. And that's where everyone must begin to rid your bodies of every disease you have. Don't drink bottled water either.

All bottled water is tap water. It has to have something in it to prevent bacteria from growing in it. If the water is pure, devoid of all the chlorine, there is nothing to prevent bacteria from thriving in that water. There are no regulations on bottled water. And when that bottled water comes to the factories where it is bottled with the chlorine already in that water, that chlorine doesn't have to be listed as an ingredient. Bottled water is only needed when your water supply badly contaminated from fracking or such.

So get those water filters – both a shower filter and a water filter. If you can't afford the $110 for the multi-stage fluoride filter I recommended, then start out with a carbon filter. They come as counter-top, faucet-end or pitcher filters. They filter out 90% of the chlorine and no fluoride. Fluoride is a smaller particle. So it requires a better filter than carbon. When you experience your "water with no taste" for the first time, you'll know how great pure water is!

Once you've got your filters, you can drink baking soda water using your pure water. Without the chemicals in your water, it is neutral; with a pH level of 7.0. Now you can add baking soda (pH 8.5) to some pure filtered water, to reverse the acidity of your body. This acidity allowed disease to form in your body. So as we get to the next step in the basic cure for all disease, let me point out that **acidity, inflammation and disease are all the same thing.**

You poison your body with sugars, animal products, chlorinated water, white flour and other chemicals. Then once your body can no longer remove those poisons as fast as they are entering your body, they begin to gather in places in your body. Once those acidic poisons begin to destroy a part of your body, a doctor calls that disease. It doesn't matter what name doctors gave the results of poisons gathering in your body. What matters is that you recognize those poisons and avoid them.

Poisons CAUSE all disease. So dealing with the CAUSE is the way to end and eliminate all diseases in your body. Technically, 20% of all disease is caused directly by germs or viruses. But until your body becomes acidic, germs and viruses have little to no consequences on your body. An immune system that is so bogged down and backed up with attempting to remove all the poisons in your food, drinks and water, sure can't protect you when germs and viruses enter your poison soaked acidic body.

So to reverse your body's acidity you have to either become an instant vegetarian or drink baking soda water. I don't have to explain to you how to eat raw produce for most of your food. But why you need to use baking soda, at about a dollar a pound, needs some scientific explaining.

I also need to dis-spell some of the misleading information everyone runs into when deciding whether or not to start drinking baking soda water. Those misleadings can be a bit confusing. Those false assumptions center around the fact that baking soda is sodium, sodium bicarbonate, and ignorance of the facts that even doctors use baking soda for cancer and dialysis patients.

Baking Soda – A Miracle cure?

Baking soda – the closest thing there is to a miracle cure. Never ever underestimate the power of baking soda! The power of baking soda will amaze you almost every time you use it. And it's absolutely true that baking soda can save your body from radiation poisoning; whether it's from bombs or radiation treatments. And although doctors use baking soda water to keep from killing almost all their radiation patients, I've never heard a one of them say they knew they were getting baking soda water. Same thing is true about dialysis patients. They are given baking soda water during dialysis.

Doctors give you baking soda water as part of their treatments without telling you. I am telling you to drink baking soda water as the scientific way of reversing the acidity of your body to rid your body of all disease. Their baking soda water costs a few hundred dollars. The baking soda water you make yourself costs about 5 cents or less for the same amount.

Baking soda ended the last disease I had, gout. My kidney disease, heart disease, arthritis, headaches, heartburn and the other 5 diseases were gone and behind me for a few years. But the gout kept coming back, until I finally found out about using baking soda for acidity in the body.

Just applying the one principle of using highly alkaline water against any kind of acid, wherever it may be, led me to the end of my gout. My thinking was "Gout is Uric ACID. Baking soda neutralizes ACID." I first drank baking soda water during a gout attack.

I would sit and do nothing as the excruciating pain of gout hammered me 24 hours a day. Then I drank some baking soda water 3 times during a gout attack. It was gone by the next morning. When it came back in a few weeks, I drank the baking soda water a few times and the attack ended before I went to bed that same day. So I drank baking soda water almost every day for a few weeks and the gout never came back.

It takes a while to completely cure yourself of gout because, by the time you have your first gout attack, Uric Acid crystals are all over the inside of your body. So once you neutralize enough gout (Uric Acid) crystals to end your gout attacks, you still have to neutralize all the Uric Acid crystals all over your body. So, you continue drinking baking soda water until you have cleaned your food, drinks and water of most of the acidic poisons; sugars, red meat, white flour and chlorinated water.

But since cleaning up your current diet is the most difficult and time consuming part of restoring your body to health and curing every disease, I will explain how you do that last. So let's finish this up about using alkaline substances such as baking soda, to reverse the acidity of your body and bring disease to an end in your body.

Remember, acidity, disease and inflammation are the same thing. Ending acidity IS ending inflammation. Ending acidity IS ending disease. By getting rid of the excess acid in your body, you are ridding your body of all disease, inflammation. Drinking baking soda water is needed until you have learned to avoid most poisons, so your body never becomes so overloaded with poisons that it shows up as diseases in your body.

You can become a vegetarian and filter your water if you want to cure yourself of all diseases. You can also drink lots of Aloe Vera Juice to slowly reverse your body's diseased acidic state. But the best way is to drink the baking soda water and clean up your food, drinks, water and personal hygiene items; as well as correcting your diet deficiencies with vitamins.

Baking soda is great for brushing your teeth, deodorant, freshening clothes, removing odors and a lot of other beneficial things. But its ability to reverse your body's acidity is by far the best benefit of baking soda water. At a pH of around 8.5, baking soda is truly medicinal gold! It is natural and safe and your body needs it. But some question whether it is safe for everyone.

Most of this about baking soda being sodium, sodium bicarbonate. But since the body needs salt, your body puts all the sodium bicarbonate to use in your body. Your CO_2 blood serum levels tell you the total bicarbonate in your blood, which includes three different bicarbonates. These are the reasons why baking soda does not raise your blood salt levels. Consuming all salts except sodium bicarbonate and sea salt will raise your salt levels. These sodiums and table salt are poison to your body. So your body only works to remove all these man-made sodiums as fast as it can.

To use baking soda safely, follow these rules: Mix ½ teaspoon baking soda in 4-6 ounces water, and drink it 2 to 5 times a day for at least 2 or 3 months or until you have no diseases at all. Drink it on an empty stomach or no sooner than an hour before or an hour after a meal, snack or sugary drink. This will prevent uncomfortable bloating. Try and drink it before you go to bed and when you first get up each day.

Drink baking soda water for your heartburn, gout and arthritis for the best and quickest relief from this inflammation/disease. There is no need to worry whether you are drinking too much baking soda water as long as any disease exists in your body. You will be drinking baking soda water as a part of your life and health for the rest of your life. The rule for using any natural things to cure yourself is to nourish your body with 2 or 3 times the normal amount for 2 or 3 months. Then keep your body healthy with maintenance doses. This means you take all these things 2 or 3 times a week from now on. Not daily.

So get your water filters and baking soda, and start drinking baking soda mixed in filtered water, as directed. Then you can correct your major diet deficiencies. Any person who is sick has deficiencies of anti-oxidants, Magnesium and Omega-3. So let's get those corrected in your next step to restoring your entire body to health to end all diseases in your body.

Correcting Your Major Diet Deficiencies

The 3 major nutrients that your body is deficient in are anti-oxidants, Magnesium and Omega-3. The only way this could not be true is if you have been taking vitamins regularly. There is not enough anti-oxidants or Magnesium in the foods you buy at the grocery store to provide you with enough of these nutrients. And since rare few people are on a proper fish diet, almost all of us are deficient in Omega-3 also. Somehow you have to correct these nutrient deficiencies.

Take 1000mg Vitamin C and 1000mg fish oil 3 to 5 times daily; which is about every 3 or 4 hours. Also take 400mg Magnesium oxide 3 times a day. Magnesium chloride would be a good second choice if you can't find the Magnesium oxide. The same is true about using Flax seed oil instead of Fish oil. You want to take all 3 of these together.

There are so many things these 3 vitamins and food substances will do for you. Vitamin C is the amount of disease removing power you have. Vitamin C removes the poisons, toxins and free radicals that cause all diseases. If you had been taking enough Vitamin C, your body would have removed enough cancer cells to keep you from having cancer. The same thing is true with colds and the flu; as well as any diseases. Vitamin C removes the cause of all diseases. So Vitamin C is essential to curing any disease.

You will benefit by taking other anti-oxidants too, like Selenium, Beta Carotene, Vitamin E, Alpha Lipoic Acid, Grape Seed Extract and others. But none of those are as cheap and ready available as Vitamin C.

Most Vitamin C you will find is going to be Ascorbic Acid. That is an acidic form of Vitamin C. The two alkaline forms of Vitamin C are Sodium Ascorbate and Calcium Ascorbate. So you would benefit more by taking one of these two alkaline forms of Vitamin C rather than the Ascorbic Acid form.

Magnesium oxide is what I prefer since it is an oxygenated form of Magnesium. Magnesium oxide (MgO) is one part magnesium, one part oxygen. All diseased cells in your body are oxygen deficient. So taking the Magnesium oxide will increase oxygen in your body, just as water ($H2O$) does. But the most powerful thing Magnesium does is insure that over 300 body metabolisms occur. Without enough Magnesium, these body metabolisms do not occur or barely ever occur. And as this deficiency persists over time, your body grows weaker and more susceptible to more and more diseases. Your body is starving for Magnesium. And once you start taking it, you begin to feel the difference.

Lack of Magnesium causes serious problems such as bladder stones, kidney stones, bones spurs and heart arrhythmia. That's why Magnesium cures bladder stones, kidney stones, bone spurs and heart arrhythmia.

Magnesium dissolves calcium to make it available for use by the body. Lack of Magnesium leaves particles of calcium available to combine with free radicals to form bladder and kidney stones and bone spurs. Magnesium also relaxes the heart to maintain proper heart rhythm, helps regulate blood sugar levels, promotes normal blood pressure, maintains normal muscle and nerve function and keeps bones strong.

Magnesium is needed for over 300 body metabolisms and is the fourth most abundant mineral in your body. About half that amount is found in your bones.

Magnesium seems to be very good at helping to prevent or improve such diseases as diabetes, hypertension and cardiovascular disease. Magnesium can also relieve migraines and tension headaches, as well as PMS discomforts like bloating, tender breasts and swelling of your upper body.

I used Magnesium oxide tablets to stop my fourth bladder stone attack in less than an hour back in 1996. I have been taking Magnesium since then and have never had another bladder stone attack after that fourth one.

The third nutrient we're all deficient in is Omega-3. This is due mainly to the fact that the savage American diet doesn't have any Omega-3 in it! Red meat and sugar don't have Omega-3 in them! Red meat does have a high level of Omega-6, but only traces of Omega-3. Salmon, tuna and mackerel are high in Omega-3; as well as the vegetable sources of Omega-3 such as Flax seed, beans, wild rice, Canola oil and Walnuts.

So to get enough Omega-3 to prevent strokes, heart attacks, Alzheimer's, other brain diseases, arthritis and more, you are going to have to take either Fish oil or Flax seed oil supplements.

You need to take at least 1000mg of Fish oil 3 to 5 times daily for 2-3 months. Then you take 1000mg 3 or 4 times a week to provide your body with the Omega-3 it needs to stay healthy.

Fish oils contain the Omega-3 fatty acids eicosapentaenoic acid (EPA) and docosahexaenoic acid (DHA); precursors of eicosanoids that are known to reduce inflammation throughout the body. Fish oil comes from the tissues of oily fish such as cod, haddock, salmon, trout, sardine, herring and mackerel. Fish oil is high in Vitamins A and D and Omega-3 fatty acids. Its most well-known benefits are in helping those with heart disease, depression and inflammatory conditions such as arthritis. Fish oil is an anti-inflammatory.

Some of the conditions that Fish oil cures, prevents or improves are depression, peptic ulcers, Alzheimer's disease, Chron's disease, Colitis, Breast Cancer, lupus and heart disease. Fish oil also improves your skin, promotes weight loss, prevents schizophrenia, eases bi-polar disorders, improves brain function, increases eye focus and much more.

The EFAs, essential fatty acids, in Fish oil fight the plaque in the brain that causes Alzheimer's. Those already afflicted with Alzheimer's disease can reduce the symptoms of Alzheimer's.

Fish oil emulsifies the plaque that clings to your artery and blood vessel walls; which causes high blood pressure, hardening of the arteries, heart attacks and strokes. It acts like a scavenger to clean your blood and make your blood flow more smoothly. It also cures arthritis by lubricating the joints and acting as an anti-inflammatory to reduce the pain and swelling associated with arthritis. Fish oil is beneficial to the pancreas and strengthens a weak pancreas. It is also a strong ally against cancer of the pancreas.

Fish oil is proven to prevent and cure breast cancer. It kills breast cancer cells as fast as chemotherapy. This is because of the high fat content in a woman's breasts; which almost every woman is seriously deficient in, due to not being on a fish diet.

All of this is science, the Laws of Physics. Poisons cause all disease. And since this is scientific fact, poisons still cause all disease when they're FDA certified "safe" AND.... when you make excuses for making yourself sick through habitual use of these "safe" poisons. And it gets easier and easier for these poisons to make you sick, once your body is acidic and weakened by your long-term nutrient deficiencies.

And although there are quite a few other things you can do to speed your healing along, the things covered in this chapter so far will do the most good for everyone with any diseases. So let's review what you need to do first.

We deal with the acidity of our body; which allowed disease. We correct our diet deficiencies. And we get a water filter and a shower filter to eliminate our biggest source of poisons, and to wash our bodies out with pure clean filtered water daily. **Nothing detoxes better than pure water.**

You can begin doing these things as soon as you get them:

- **Drink ½ teaspoon baking soda in 4-6 oz. filtered water 3-5x daily**
- **Take 250-400mg Magnesium oxide 3 to 4 times daily**
- **1000mg Vitamin C 3 to 5 times daily, and**
- **1000mg Fish oil (and/or flax seed oil) 3 times daily**

And once you have your shower and water filters, you:

- **Drink 1-ounce pure water for every 2 pounds body weight daily**

That's how easy it is to restore your body to health. But unless you do all these things and become an instant vegetarian you are not going to rid your body of all disease. You absolutely WILL cure yourself of a lot of diseases. But since the majority of poisons that cause your diseases are in your food and drinks, you have to learn how to clean up your diet to reduce those poisons to cure yourself of all disease. You can't totally eliminate all poisons.

You have to stop poisoning yourself in order to completely cure yourself and keep any disease from returning. After all, you made yourself sick by eating so much poison that it made you sick. Now you have to find out what those poisons are, and stop eating and drinking them.

Improving the quality of your food and drinks is not an easy thing to do, and also takes a while to learn how to do. But in one of the next chapters I will teach you how to avoid the most poisons and the worst poisons in your food, drinks and water. But before I get to cleaning up your diet, there are some things you need to know that will help. By focusing on restoring your body to health, instead of trying different things for each and every disease you have, you are on the path to ending all diseases.

Having a constant supply of pure water going into my body still gives me joy every time I drink it! There is no detox better than the constant washing of the inside of your body with filtered water that is PURE H2O!

When someone asks me how to cure cancer, I tell them to start by doing the things just stated in this book – getting the water filters, drinking pure water and baking soda water and taking Magnesium, Vitamin C and Fish Oil. And when someone asks me the cure for kidney disease, heart disease or any disease, it's still the same things you must do to cure those diseases and any diseases.

So do these things as the foundation for restoring your body to health.

I never set out to cure myself of my chronic kidney disease. And I never even thought about any possibility of me curing my gout, arthritis, bleeding intestines and gums, headaches, heartburn or any other disease. But that's what I did. I cured myself of every disease I had. But all I was trying to do was add some time to my life, after doctors said I would be on dialysis or dead within 2 or 3 years. That meant by 2008 or 2009.

If I had someone to teach me these things to cure myself, OR just tell me WATCH WHAT YOU DRINK, I could have cured myself in 1/5 the time. I also might have avoided any kidney failure altogether. I had to dig my way out of the hole I dug myself into while hearing nothing but "there's no cure for kidney disease" and "there's no reversing kidney disease".

But that's what the medical profession says about ALL diseases. That's why 150,000,000 Americans are permanently sick. Because doctors REFUSE to cure anyone. All cures are OUTSIDE doctors and their medical profession. And there is NO CONNECTION between cures and doctors.

They don't mind telling you to stop smoking and drinking or change your diet. But they never do anything to cure anyone. So it's all up to YOU to use science to cure yourself naturally like about 85% of Americans did up until they patented their first chemical "medicine" in 1939.

And since it's not possible to get any help from doctors when we want to cure ourselves, there's no use pretending you will. It's between your mind and body, and science. Your body can heal itself if you nourish it properly and stop bombarding it with poison after poison each and every day.

If you hadn't consumed so much acidic foods, drinks and water, you wouldn't need to reverse the acidity they caused. And you wouldn't have the diseases those poisons cause once your body is acidic.

Acidic cells have less oxygen than healthy cells. A cell becomes cancerous once it has lost 35% of its oxygen. Raising the pH of your body, by neutralizing acid, causes the oxygen levels in cells to increase. You make it hard to raise your body's pH when you continue bombarding it with poisons while you are trying to heal it.

Your body just has a certain amount of energy. That energy is best spent on repairing damaged cells. But the more acidic your body is, the less energy it has to repair damaged cells. It has to spend its energy on removing all those poisons in your shower and drinking water, food, drinks, personal hygiene items and all other sources, before it has a chance to. Not only does this waste valuable energy, these poisons do damage until they are removed.

You can't beat science or get around it. The Laws of Physics that dictate the health of your body are what you must learn. I am using this next chapter to give you some quick cures to some diseases, using the sciences I have shared with you so far in this book. I will also tell you how these sciences cure these diseases.

I have come to believe that the quality of your health is equal to the quality of your water. You need pure water to pump life into your entire body. That water cannot contain bacteria destroying chlorine! The main item you need to cure yourself is a filter for your shower and drinking water.

But if you just want to know the cure for all disease in as few a words as possible, here's a graphic I use to sum up all you have to do to restore your entire body to health in order to cure yourself of all diseases; and maintain those cures and excellent health.

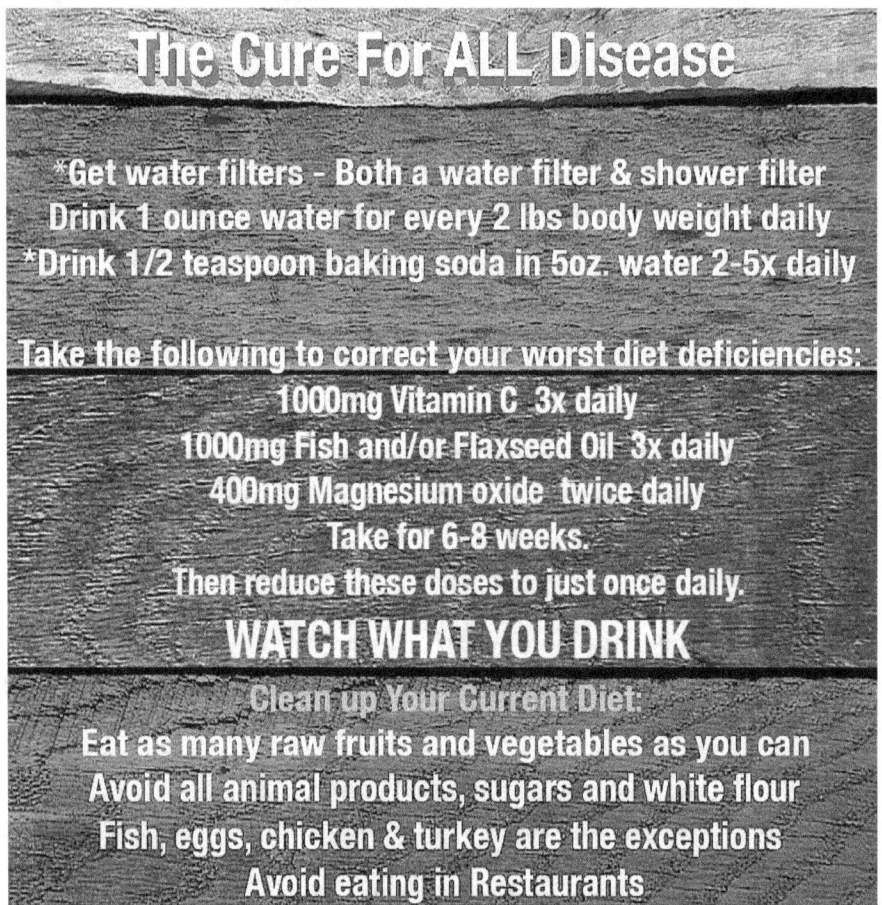

The Cure For ALL Disease

*Get water filters - Both a water filter & shower filter
Drink 1 ounce water for every 2 lbs body weight daily
*Drink 1/2 teaspoon baking soda in 5oz. water 2-5x daily

Take the following to correct your worst diet deficiencies:
1000mg Vitamin C 3x daily
1000mg Fish and/or Flaxseed Oil 3x daily
400mg Magnesium oxide twice daily
Take for 6-8 weeks.
Then reduce these doses to just once daily.
WATCH WHAT YOU DRINK
Clean up Your Current Diet:
Eat as many raw fruits and vegetables as you can
Avoid all animal products, sugars and white flour
Fish, eggs, chicken & turkey are the exceptions
Avoid eating in Restaurants

So let's get to those cures that can bring you great relief very quickly, if you know why certain sciences cure certain diseases so effectively.

3 - Some Easy Quick Cures

What I have told you so far will cure you of almost every disease you have, but will not keep you cured of all disease unless you learn to recognize and avoid the saturation of poisons in your food, drinks, water and other sources.

There are some diseases that you can cure by just drinking baking soda water OR just taking Magnesium OR just taking Fish Oil. So to make sure you get relief as quickly as possible, I am going to tell you some quick cures for some diseases. I have to tell you this because the first major disease I cured myself of was achieved by just doing one of these items I told you to take. That item was Magnesium oxide.

In 1996, I had my third bladder stone attack. I had to go to the ER and ran up a few thousand dollars in medical bills in that one visit. When I got all the bills for that visit I called the doctor from the ER and told him I had no problem paying the bills as long as he would tell me how to cure myself of bladder stones. I told him I could pay these bills, but could not afford to pay these amounts every time I had an attack; which was about one a year so far.

His staff started threatening to call the Police if I didn't stop asking them how to cure bladder stones. I told them that was fine as long as they told me how to cure myself of bladder stones too. That's when they started claiming I was the devil and did so repeatedly. I then told them several times "OK, I'm the devil and you're going to call the Police. So just tell me how to cure myself of these bladder stones and I won't ever bother you again."

After going back and forth like this for 10 or 15 minutes with the doctor and his staff, the doctor finally told me the only thing I could do is to drink lots of water. He said that would help pass the bladder stones quicker. But he never gave me a cure. So I kept my word and never paid the bills.

But my sweet little CockaPoo suffered with many bladder stones for 8 or 10 years until she died a few years at the age of 18 years old. I was devastated but obsessed with never letting that happen again. I searched and searched for a solution to bladder stones. And I thought I knew what would prevent them if any of my future dogs ever had them.

It was that information I finally remembered when I was in the middle of my fourth bladder stone attack. I told my wife it was a waste of time to go back to the ER. I also told her I couldn't take this pain. And when I went and laid down to try and endure this hopeless situation, I remembered what I had learned from our CockaPoo having bladder stones.

So I told my wife to see if we had any Magnesium. We did. So I took 2 250mg Magnesium oxide tablets. Less than an hour later the attack stopped. I took the little strainer I got from my visit to the ER and peed through it the rest of the day to see if I could see any stones. But I never saw any. And I never had another bladder stone attack since then.

I realized the Magnesium had dissolved the Calcium that makes up the largest portion of bladder stones, and had done that so well that there were no stones left in my bladder. Not even any little pieces! And that was my first experience with curing chronic disease.

Bladder stones, as well as kidney stones and bone spurs, are formed by particles of Calcium combining with poisons/free radicals to form these prickly stones. So by taking a large dose of Magnesium oxide on an empty stomach, all that Magnesium dissolved those Calcium particles in my bladder stones. This destroyed the bladder stones.

If you take the Magnesium along with Vitamin C, you make it impossible for bladder stones and bone spurs to exist in your body. The Magnesium dissolves the Calcium so it is not available to form stones. The Vitamin C removes the toxins/free radicals which make up the rest of your stones.

At the time I cured myself of bladder stones, I had headaches, heartburn and arthritis most days. I also had intestinal bleeding and bleeding gums. So this is why I know you can cure yourself of bladder stones and other diseases without doing all the things I've told you to do so far.

It wasn't until my kidneys were saturated with poisons and failed that I discovered how to cure all diseases. I realized I had discovered the cure for all disease after I cured myself of every disease I had. Yes, AFTER, not before or during! And I had to do it without any help from anyone.

Those of you who choose to cure yourselves will be pretty much all alone in doing so. I am certain of you being cured with science. But that's because I have been as sick as you can be and cured myself of every disease I had. Most of the diseases I had, I didn't ever put any thought or effort into curing any of them. Everything was about helping my kidneys in hopes I could add some time to my life. Nothing else!

I didn't take Fish oil for my arthritis. I took it to see if it would help my kidneys. Everything I took was to try and help my kidneys. It was after I had sustained a reversal of my kidney disease for 2 or 3 years that I finally realized I had cured myself of every disease I had.

Regardless of how strange that may seem to some, I told you so you would realize how obsessed I was with helping my kidneys. No one ever said I could die from headaches, heartburn, arthritis or dandruff. It was kidney disease that almost killed me several times and would end up killing me soon if I didn't last long enough to have a successful kidney transplant. They still cost in excess of $262,000 in the first year too.

I tried a lot of stuff that didn't help and at least one thing that almost killed me. That was from an Australian guy's PDF sold online at those web sites made specifically to sell this one scam. He had these 3 or 4 separate set of instructions, depending on what caused your kidney disease. It was natural stuff. So I believed it would be safe. But it wasn't. But before you get scared of doing natural things, let me tell you what happened.

His plan included doing 600mg Alpha Lipoic Acid a day until cured. As I started this, my doctor warned me not to take 600mg a day. I told him I would take it until it caused problems. About 2 and a half months later my Potassium was up to 5.6. My doctor said this is what he warned me about.

Alpha Lipoic Acid not only causes your kidneys to reuse nutrients like Vitamin C up to 3 or 4 times, it also causes your kidneys to reuse Potassium repeatedly. This is dangerous. Once I stopped taking the 600mg of Alpha Lipoic Acid, my Potassium went down to just 4.8 three weeks later.

If I had continued doing the 600mg of Alpha Lipoic Acid, my Potassium would have continued to climb and resulted in severe heart problems. I could have easily died from heart palpitations.

Why this Australian man could tell anyone to take these high doses of Alpha Lipoic Acid for more than 6-8 weeks maximum, is quite irresponsible.

You won't ever see me telling you to take mega doses of anything for more than 2-3 months at a time. And when I say 2-3 months, I mean for you to take it for two months and for you to decide when to stop the mega doses during the third month. Any longer than that is a decision you have to make for yourself without my approval.

This is because we are just taking mega doses at first to make up for the huge amounts of acid in your body and severe deficiencies of major nutrients like Magnesium, Omega-3 and anti-oxidants like Vitamin C. Once you have done that for at least 2 months, you just need the RDA. You will need to take these things 2 or 3 times a week for the rest of your life to stay healthy. Your failure to do this in the first place, resulted in your body becoming weak and far more susceptible to the effects of acid and the diseases it brings.

The results you get from doing these things and cleaning up the huge amounts of poisons in your food, drinks, water and other sources, is that you rid your body of ALL diseases.

But regardless of whether you do all it takes to restore your entire body to health and rid it of all diseases, here are some quick cures:

Arthritis – Fish oil

Bladder stones – Magnesium; and Vitamin C

Bone spurs – Magnesium; and Vitamin C

Dandruff and Dry hair – shower filter

Dry itchy skin – shower filter

Gout – baking soda water

Heartburn – baking soda water
Heart arrhythmia - Magnesium
Kidney stones – Magnesium; and Vitamin C
Uric Acid kidney stones – baking soda water; Magnesium and Vitamin C
Migraines – Magnesium

Fish oil lubricates your joints and fights inflammation.
Magnesium dissolves Calcium and Vitamin C removes toxins.
Shower filters remove the chlorine that drys your skin, scalp and hair.
Baking soda water neutralizes gout (Uric Acid crystals)
….and neutralizes stomach acid.
Magnesium relaxes your heart to create proper heart rhythm.
Baking soda water dissolves Uric acid stones.
Migraines are caused by muscle tension from a Magnesium deficiency.
So reach for the Magnesium instead of the pain pills and pacemakers.

You can apply these scientific principles to more and more metabolisms in your body and see how Magnesium, baking soda, Vitamin C, Fish oil and pure water are such vital necessities for our bodies.

Magnesium also lowers blood pressure by relaxing your heart and creating and maintaining proper heart rhythm. The most powerful fact about taking Magnesium is how it is needed for over 300 body metabolisms. And the less Magnesium your body has, the less those metabolisms will occur.

All of you use water to wash your dishes, clothes, cars, babies, bodies and most everything else. But when it comes to telling people to wash the INSIDE of their body with water, people just don't seem to understand why or how that could be so important. But it IS. And it's NUMBER ONE on the list!

Wash your bodies out with pure filtered water. Do not drink lots of water that still has all the chlorine in it! That does as much damage as it does good.

Wash, detox, your body by drinking 1-ounce pure filtered water for every two pounds of body weight each day. And make that a change for life.

Not only does pure filtered water wash your insides, your body is 80% water, H2O, not H2O+chlorine+fluoride.

This helps alkalize your body. And the oxygen gives life to your body.

Someone with COPD, pulmonary fibrosis or any other lung disease is down right crazy to NOT have a shower filter and multi-stage fluoride filter. All that chlorine going in your body killing the oxygen in every cell it comes in contact with, while you struggle for every breath! It's unbelievable how blind people choose to be about how harmful poisons really are!

One fellow asked me if I knew how to cure high blood pressure caused by excess salt. I told him, yes, stop eating and drinking all those products with sodiums in them. He asked if there was anyway to cure his HBP without doing without those sodium packed products. And of course the answer is No! You cannot get rid of any problem without getting rid of the CAUSE of that problem. And POISONS CAUSE ALL DISEASES.

Even though the CDC says around 20% of all disease is caused by germs and viruses, fact is that only a rare few germs or viruses can spread in your body unless it is already weakened by major long term nutrient deficiencies and/or being in an acidic state from consuming sugars, white flour, animal products and chlorinated water.

And even though poisons cause all disease, doctors give you their poison chemical drugs that your body works to remove the instant you take it. And it works until it removes all those prescription drugs from your body.

Your body only has a certain amount of energy. And you need to use as much of that energy as possible to repair damaged cells.

Your body is diseased from excess poisons accumulating in parts of your body. You continue poisoning yourself at the same rate. So where is your body going to get the energy to heal itself?

You have to stop eating as much food, and avoid the worst poisons that are in sodas, juices and other sugary flavored drinks. But no one tells you to WATCH WHAT YOU DRINK! And that's how I blew out my kidneys.

You have to focus on the total amount of poisons that are entering your body. That includes smoking, drinking alcohol, street drugs, aspirin, Tylenol, Advil, Aleve, garden chemicals, exposure in work places, soaps, shampoo, lotions, deodorants, lipstick, make up and a wide array of other places.

Add to that, all the poisons in your food, drinks and water, and you can see how massively you are poisoning your body every day.

You wake up in the morning. Saturate your entire body with chlorinated water that soaks into every pore, while you breath chlorinated gas in the steamy hot shower. Scrub your body with chemical soap. Shampoo with chemical shampoo. Then rub on the chemical underarm deodorant.

Then you eat your mostly poison white biscuits with greasy gravy. Add 3 or 4 slices of dead pig flesh. And a cup of coffee with sugar and chlorinated water. Then you at least had some eggs, which are good for you. But you saturated them in grease to cook them.

Then you have lunch in a restaurant. You have a hamburger and soda. That's drug drenched red meat on a pure poison white bun. And 12-ounces of an acidic beverage with a pH of 3.5, 4-Tablespoons of gene mutating high fructose corn syrup made from genetically altered corn in a 3 step process using genetically altered enzymes. It will take your immune system 6 hours to completely remove the poisons in that one 12-ounce soda. And that is after it has done lots of damage to your insides.

Then you still have dinner. You might have more drug saturated red meat and some potatoes. And some iced tea. If it's sugary, then the potatoes are the only thing that is good for you.

You have a snack later on. Then it's bed time shortly after the snack, to sleep 7 or 8 hours, then begin all of this for the next day; and the next day.

After years of all this daily poisoning, your body has become acidic. That is when the poisons begin to accumulate in parts of your body and get named by your doctor as some disease.

So it's not just what you eat that determines how many diseases you have. But the total amount of poisons that enter your body.

Drinking the baking soda water is a temporary solution to reversing the acidity of your body. But the real solution is to stop poisoning your body with these poisons, to stop the cause of all diseases.

That is the complicated and difficult part of curing yourself and maintaining those cures. What we have covered so far is pretty simple.

So in the next chapter I will tell you how to clean up your current diet, drinks and personal hygiene items, to insure that you maintain your cures.

It doesn't matter what names doctors gave your diseases. They will all be gone by using scientific Laws of Physics that dictate the health of our bodies.

Let the graphic at the end of Chapter 2 be your simple guide to restoring your body to health to rid it of all disease. But use this next chapter to clean up your diet. Corporations use a lot of deceit in their labeling.

So let's get to the complicated part of all this. Corporations are never going to remove the drugs they put in their foods and drinks to addict you to those products. So it's up to YOU to find those poisons and avoid them.

4 - Avoiding the Poisons That Cause All Diseases

Poisons cause all diseases. Even the 20% of diseases that are said to be caused by germs and viruses, couldn't spread in your body without your body being acidic from habitual poisoning. Eliminate most poisons from entering your body and your immune system can easily fight any germs or bacteria before they spread and become a disease.

You could be a vegetarian. But unless you watch what you drink, what you drink will make you sick and kill you! And this plague has become so bad that 90% of the US population dies from disease; with 95% of those deaths being blamed on the saturation of poisons in our food, drinks and water.

But all disease is caused by the total amount of poisons entering your body and the toxicity of those poisons. And the most poisons entering your body usually do enter in your food and drinks. So although cleaning up your diet will do an immense amount of good for your body, only a few ever cure themselves merely by changing their diet.

A cigarette smoker needs to stop inhaling the pure poison smoke, not to mention the tar, nicotine and other poisons. Same with alcohol. You have to reduce the amount of cigarettes you smoke and the amount of alcohol you drink. But you also need that shower filter and water filter; and those Vitamins and Fish oil to correct your diet deficiencies.

You also need to back off the Aspirin, Ibuprofen, Aleve, Tylenol, heartburn pills and any and all over-the-counter medications. And once you have made a habit of nourishing your body properly and stopped the massive poisoning of your body, you won't have the need or desire for any of that stuff!

You also have almost pure poison chemical shampoo, soap, deodorant, all your make up, lotions, hair color, hair spray, toothpaste, mouthwash and a host of other chemicals you use on your body. Your pores soak up these poisons the entire time you are using them.

It's all these poisons combined, the total amount, that determines when your body develops disease. Taking Vitamin C and other anti-oxidants will remove these disease-causing poisons, but only after they have already done a lot of damage. **Not allowing these poisons to enter your body in the first place is the real solution to curing and preventing all disease.**

And of course, that begins with drinking pure water; free of chlorine, fluoride and any other poisons or impurities in your water. I can never say it enough about how PURE water is the most precious thing you can possibly put into your body.

I tell everyone to drink PURE FILTERED water. If your water is not filtered, don't drink very much of it. Not only do water and shower filters filter out the poisons in your water, water is one-third oxygen and washes, detoxes, your insides. Your body doesn't have to be damaged or spend energy removing all those poisons if you use filters. But once you have your water and shower filters, you still drink other things besides water. So let me give you some tips and insight that will help you and your family reduce the amount of poisons in what you drink, until you have found healthy replacements.

WATCH WHAT YOU DRINK!

If only someone had told me this, my kidneys wouldn't have failed when they did, and I might have avoided kidney failure altogether. But all anyone talks about is watch what you eat. And I ate as healthy as anyone I knew. My diet was extremely good and included thousands of dollars of Organic food that we have grown since 1982.

When my kidneys failed, no doctor could tell me what caused that. They did tell me that high blood pressure caused my kidney failure. But what caused my blood pressure to shoot up to 240/140 and stay there for months; blowing my kidneys out in the process? I got no answers from anyone. And what caused my blood pressure to skyrocket was not something I found out until a few years later on my own.

Your liver converts excess sugars to bad cholesterol, LDL. It is this reason why excess sugar gives you high blood pressure. Excess sugars also cause diabetes due to your body's inability to convert excessive amounts of sugar into energy. Your pancreas is overworked by all the energy it has to spend producing insulin to convert sugars to energy, and producing excessive amounts of enzymes to digest all the food you failed to chew up and cover with your saliva before swallowing.

When these sugars are in liquid form, lots of bad things happen in your body. Sugars in liquids are digested faster and absorbed into your bloodstream much quicker. Your body also puts more of the sugars in liquids to use than in solid foods. On a positive note, this is also why juicing is great.

Since everyone is blind to the massive damage and diseases you get from what you drink, you have to start from scratch when trying to figure out what you can drink that is healthy. Then when you learn that corporations don't sell anything in grocery stores that is healthy, you seek to learn if there's anything you can drink that is NOT poisonous. And just as it is with all food, you end up having to learn which drinks are the least poisonous.

Unless you drink pure filtered water and make your own juices from fresh produce, there will be lots of poison in everything you drink.

Make unsweetened tea with tap water, no water filter, and you swig down all that chlorine, fluoride, dozens of other chemicals, dirt and debris; which your body has to work to remove it all. Same with 100% of the things you drink that are made with water.

Since I can't really tell you any non-poisonous drinks, I'm going to tell you how to clean up your current drinks. That includes some nice variations to what you are currently drinking, the least poisonous and most poisonous products you can buy. Almost 100% of the drinks you can buy are just flavored sugar waters. So let's take a look at sugars.

Sugars

This includes white granulated sugar, brown sugar, pure cane sugar, fructose, high fructose corn syrup, honey and more.

Out of all the sugars and sweeteners there are, only brown pure cane sugar, raw honey and Stevia are not pure poison. Brown pure cane sugar is not healthy, but is far less toxic than white granulated sugar. Stick to these sugars for sweeteners to minimize the levels of toxins in your drinks; and also in your food. High fructose corn syrup is by far the worst poison of all.

High fructose corn syrup is made with genetically altered corn in a 3-step process using genetically altered enzymes. White granulated sugar is made by removing everything of nutritional value from sugar cane and heating that to 1000 degrees 3 times. Brown sugar is just white granulated sugar sprayed with molasses. Raw honey is the only honey that is not as bad as sugar.

Raw honey is cloudy, not clear like Honey Bear honey. Raw honey would have to be on grocery shelves directly from local bee farmers, since shelf life is only about 3 months. After then, it would become a solid.

Brown pure cane sugar is the sugar cane before you process out all the nutritional value of the sugar cane to begin making white granulated sugar. It is then dried to be sold in dry powder/crystal form rather than liquid form. So this makes brown pure cane sugar the most natural mass marketed sugar. You can buy Zulka Pure Cane Sugar at Wal-Mart.

Stevia is an herb that is about 30 times as sweet as sugar. Stevia can be used to sweeten tea and many other beverages. We use Stevia to sweeten our Lipton tea. Everyone tells me that Stevia doesn't taste sweet. This is because it doesn't give them that "sugar burn" you get from white sugar and high fructose corn syrup. But Stevia is sweet.

Just make some Lipton tea and put a few ounces of it aside unsweetened. Then add the Stevia to the remainder of the tea. Taste the Stevia sweetened tea, then the unsweetened tea. Ah ha! It IS sweet. And this is exactly how I eliminated at least 150 POUNDS of sugar in liquid form every year!

Use raw honey to sweeten any small amounts of things you drink, like cups of herbal tea, coffee or glass of tea. Using raw honey as one-for-one sugar substitutes in not a practical thing to do and becomes very expensive.

Now that you know how to have something to drink that's not all poison, let's look at the things to drink that are common to almost everyone of us. That would be soda pops, fruit juices and milks.

High Fructose Corn Syrup

The most damaging poison of all is high fructose corn syrup. Since high fructose corn syrup is the most damaging poison of all, in both food and drinks, you need to know why this is a fact. So before we go on with more about what you drink, let's take a closer look at the #1 poison in our food and drinks – high fructose corn syrup.

It is not only the most toxic chemical, there is more high fructose corn syrup in our food and drinks than any other man-made UN-natural substance in your food and drinks. Corporations deliberately addict you to their poisons to make you crave their products.

Fructose is pleasing to your brain, since fructose in found in all fruits. And by increasing the amount of fructose in what you eat and drink, this tricks your mind into accepting high fructose corn syrup as pleasing. You stuff your face with foods and drinks saturated with high fructose corn syrup whether you are 100 pounds overweight or skinny as a bean pole.

Your mind has become addicted to that powerful drug called high fructose corn syrup. Now when I see a fat person, I no longer see them as lazy and pathetic. I see a poor soul with a high fructose corn syrup addiction. And until you realize that addiction WHILE you are eating and drinking products saturated with sugar and high fructose corn syrup, that addiction will continue to destroy your health as you get fatter and fatter.

Besides all my personal experiences in learning how true this mind addiction is, I have found scientists who have confirmed this scientifically.

The HMF in high fructose corn syrup, hydroxymethylfurfural, has been linked to DNA damage in humans. HMF content rises as high fructose corn syrup gets warm. Once it reaches 120 degrees Fahrenheit, HMF levels rise dramatically; regardless of the product containing high fructose corn syrup.

Then in early 2012, I learned of some long-awaited scientific backing of what I already believed to be true, when I happened to catch a CBS episode of 60 Minutes. I saw them advertise that program and didn't want to watch it because I knew they would just say how stupid all of us are for saying anything bad about sugar, and especially that sick crap known as high fructose corn syrup.

My wife and I watched the show, knowing what they were gonna do. The only hope was that Dr. Sanjay Gupta was hosting the segment. I kept the remote in my hand, ready to turn it, to keep from hearing their nonsense. But as it turns out, I got a big surprise from that segment.

Dr. Robert Lustig of the University of California at San Francisco is called a pioneer in what some call "the war against sugar". The main diseases Dr. Lustig says are linked to sugar are type II Diabetes, Obesity, Hypertension and Heart disease. He says the American lifestyle is killing us and at least 75% of it is preventable. Dr. Lustig has published at least a dozen articles on the evils of sugar. But the way most people heard what he had to say was through his video on You Tube called Sugar: The Bitter Truth. Dr. Lustig and I are in agreement on everything except one point.

He says high fructose corn syrup is no worse than any other sugar. He does admit that it's the fructose that we crave, because there is fructose in every fruit; but not in the high amounts as in high fructose corn syrup. And in fruits, that fructose is diluted by water, fiber and nutrients. That's why consuming fructose in fruits is the way to have a balanced diet. But when we consume high fructose corn syrup, it doesn't seem bad at all, since we were born to love fructose, in all our fruits, naturally.

In that same report, they told about a nutritional biologist at the University of California Davis, who conducted a 5-year study linking excessive high fructose corn syrup consumption to diseases such as heart disease and stroke. Her study showed that calories from high fructose corn syrup effected the body differently than calories from other sources. She used a completely controlled environment in her study.

Her subjects were in a kind of 24- hour a day lockdown. Everything they ate was weighed and calories counted. They began eating normal meals, then began adding sugar in their diets so that 25% of their calories were from sugar. And in just two weeks, the ones who got 25% of their calories from high fructose corn syrup, had higher levels of bad cholesterol, LDL and other increased indicators of cardiovascular disease.

What they discovered was that when your liver gets overloaded with fructose, it begins converting it to fat, which produces LDL; which forms the plaque that clogs your arteries and blood vessels.

Their report also included some information on research studying the effects of sugar, glucose, on cancer cells. Cancer cells feed and grow by hijacking the flow of glucose in your blood stream. This is especially true with cancers known to have insulin receptors. And then there was the guy who did CAT scans on the brains of humans to see the effects of high fructose corn syrup on the brain.

He found out that high fructose corn syrup affects the brain in the same way as cocaine does. Dr. Sanjay Gupta volunteered to have the CAT scans done while he was given a sip of soda pop through a tube. The CAT scan showed blood flow increased to certain parts of the brain as the soda hit his tongue. His brain began to release dopamine, as though it was some kind of addictive drug. The person conducting these tests on hundreds of people is Eric Stice, a Neuro Scientist at the Oregon Research Institute.

He concluded that as you eat more and more sugar, your body builds a tolerance to it. That causes you to crave more and more sugar as this tolerance level increases over time. This is exactly what happens when you are addicted to drugs. And that brings me to the strangest part of that segment. Actually it was the only strange part to me.

At one point, Dr. Sanjay Gupta is talking to this Dr. Lustig, the guy they said was leading the war on sugar. Sanjay asks Dr. Lustig if he is going to go out on a limb and say that sugar is a toxin, a poison. Well, Dr. Lustig said he believes it is. But what about ME? I didn't go out on a limb recently and say sugar is a poison. No, that was Dr. Lustig.

I'm the guy who not only went out on a limb and said sugar is a poison, I said white granulated sugar is a drug. I didn't go out on a limb saying that. I rode a rocket ship off THAT limb. And I rode a rocket ship off that limb back at least 30 years ago; about 1981.

I was really thrilled to see this doctor and these scientists presenting solid scientific evidence to back up what I began saying 30 years ago. It was high fructose corn syrup in sodas and fruit juices that blew out my kidneys in 2006; not to mention all the sugared tea and Gatorade I also drank daily.

So let's start with one of the most toxic product you can drink, soda pops.

Soda pops

Most soda pops are sweetened with about 4-Tablespoons of highly toxic high fructose corn syrup; as well as containing DNA-altering sodium benzoate, DNA-altering HMF and an acidity of between 3.0 and 3.5.

Problem is, that your body's pH needs to be between 6.0 and 7.3. The further below 7.3 you get, the more your pH adversely affects and impedes body metabolisms. In simple words, drinking sodas makes your body ripe for disease just because of the extreme acidity.

Then add to that, the sodium benzoate that has been proven to have the ability to switch off vital parts of DNA in a cell's mitochondria. And when you add Vitamin C in with the sodium benzoate it produces benzene, a known carcinogenic substance. The mitochondria is called the power station of the DNA. So this damage is severe and leads to serious cell malfunction. This damage is linked to such diseases as Parkinson's and Alzheimer's disease, many neuro-degenerative diseases and most of all, the whole aging process.

I went from drinking at least one thousands sodas a year to somewhere around 10 to 12 sodas a year. As I look back at this, I have no doubt as to why my kidneys failed. All these serious poisons, not to mention the fact that one 12-ounce soda pop shuts down your immune system for about 6 hours.

Technically it does not shut your immune system down. It takes about six hours to remove all the ingredients in one 12-ounce soda. Drink a soda every 6 hours and you, in essence, have no immune system working to protect you. How do you have a chance against sickness in this condition!

By drinking sodas that contain man-made sweeteners like Aspartame, Sucralose, Saccharin and others, you are consuming some very dangerous chemicals. And besides the danger of these chemical sweeteners, you still have all the other chemicals and a 3.0 acidity in every soda.

Aspartame is some bad crap! Just the fact that Aspartame turns to formaldehyde at about 80 degrees is plenty reason to avoid it. Aspartame is made up of Phenylalanine, aspartic acid and methanol. Your body converts methanol into formaldehyde. Phenylalanine and aspartic acid directly affect the brain and central nervous system and help create mood disorders, memory loss and neurological problems.

Sucralose is the sweetener family name for a brand named product called Splenda. Sucralose is created by chlorinating sugar. The chemical structure of the chlorine used in creating Sucralose is the same as the banned chemical DDT. Avoiding all these man-made sweeteners is advice everyone should heed. Another one is Saccharin.

Saccharin is a sulfa-based sweetener whose main ingredient is benzoic sulfimide. But although Saccharin is the most investigated of all the artificial sweeteners, people tend to believe it can cause bladder cancer, diarrhea, allergies and skin problems. But it seems to be the safest one. I'm not aware of any mass-marketed drinks that contain Saccharin. But I wanted to mention it, in case there are some on the market.

The safest soda pop I have found is Sierra Mist Natural. It's a lemon lime soda that, believe it or not, does not contain high fructose corn syrup or man-made artificial sweeteners. It just contains sugar. The ingredients are carbonated water, sugar, citric acid, natural flavor and potassium citrate. Citric acid is organic.

Potassium citrate is a potassium salt of citric acid. Sugar is a processed food substance and carbonated water is water that has had carbon dioxide gas under pressure dissolved in it. So that's a pretty good soda, except for the acidic carbonated water and the empty calories of the sugar.

But it doesn't have a yucky chemical taste to it compared to sodas with high fructose corn syrup and sodium benzoate. That's a tremendous improvement over all other sodas. So I'll be drinking a few of them. I'll be splitting them with my wife since I only drink half a can at a time nowadays.

If you look hard enough you can find some sodas with pure cane sugar. If you gotta have a soda, these are the least harmful, like Sierra Mist. If you can't resist drinking sodas, at least reduce the amount you drink. And make as many of those Sierra Mist, or other soda free of high fructose corn syrup and man-made artificial sweeteners.

Fruit Juices

When you begin cleaning up the saturation of poisons in your drinks, you find out that all those juices you've been drinking are almost as bad for you as sodas. They aren't as acidic and don't have DNA-altering sodium benzoate. But they have as much high fructose corn syrup and sugar as sodas do. And since it's all in liquid form, you have to try and avoid them much more than sugary foods.

Every time you drink a soda or some fruit juice you get an instant buzz, which we all think is a quick energy boost. But a lot of that feeling is really your body going to war trying to protect itself from that flood of poisons you just poured into your body. The first evidence of this is that burning of your mouth, gums and throat. This causes your mouth to become dry.

Food and drinks are for nourishing the body, not for giving your body sensations. And since no one can stop us from habitually harming ourselves this way, we all just eat and drink our way to sickness. We refuse to face the reality that what we ate and drank that we loved so much, has brought us the result of sickness; chronic sickness.

So what fruit juices are safe enough to drink? Well, you have to sift through all the deceitful labeling first. The most deceitful ones are the FDA definition of concentrate and claiming it's "100% fruit juice".

Concentrate is not juice that is boiled down to be more concentrated. No! The FDA definition allows corporations to pack as much sugar in concentrate as they choose. No "concentrate" is really concentrated fruit juice. It has some in it, but isn't the main ingredient. These facts are on their labels.

The same is true with their fraudulent term "100% Fruit Juice". Just seeing in the ingredients that there is more than just fruit juice confirms how false this term is. If it's Apple juice and it really is "100% fruit juice", then the ONLY ingredient would be Apple juice. Finding a fruit juice that is only fruit juice is a pretty frustrating task. Musselman's Apple juice is one. And some of the orange juices are decent choices.

With orange juices you just have to look for the ones that say "Not from concentrate" and "Never from concentrate". Then check to see if it has any ingredients listed. If a product says it's Orange Juice and has nothing in it BUT orange juice, you won't see any ingredients listed. The problem with even the best orange juice products is that they are stored in underground vats for months before being taken to market.

Your best choices are Simply Orange, Florida Nature and Tropicana orange juices. But always read their labels before buying, since most companies love to change what's in their products without telling you.

This is the best you can do for fruit juice, besides buying your own juicer and making your own fresh fruit juices. Although investing $100 or more in a quality juicer may not set well with you at first, just think of all that pure naturally sweetened juice you and your family will be drinking. And not a drop of it with any white sugars, high fructose corn syrup or chemical sweeteners.

It was Ocean Spray juices that played a main role in almost killing me. I drank a quart a day. It was mostly cranberry and varieties of cranberry and their other fruit juices that I drank for about 5 years daily. And all that time I thought I was drinking something healthy. But it all had more high fructose corn syrup in it than soda pops do.

Regardless of what drink you buy, almost all drinks are just flavored sugar water. That alone is enough to know to avoid them. But once you eliminate all the sodas and fruit juices that are saturated with poisons, about all that is left is vegetable juice and milk.

You might enjoy herbal teas too, unsweetened, or sweetened with a teaspoon or two of raw honey. There are a lot of herbal teas. I'll tell you about some of the best herbal teas. But first, let's see about milk.

Milk – Whole, 2%, Skim, Soy or what?

When I was dying of chronic kidney disease and had realized how bad sodas and fruit juices are, I was wondering what poisons I was gonna find in my milk that would leave me with nothing to drink but filtered water. I tried switching to 2% milk. But it tasted weak to me. While I went back and forth between whole milk and 2% milk, I researched the information about the various types of milk.

Whole milk is at least 3.25% milk fat. 2% milk is 2% milk fat. And skim and non-fat milk contain no more than 0.5% milk fat by weight. The significance of the fat content is that the growth hormones, antibiotics and other chemicals are concentrated and stored in fat cells in mammals; which includes cattle and humans. So the more fat in the milk, the more of these drugs and chemicals you will be consuming.

When you try switching from whole milk to a lower fat milk, you will probably have a hard time and want to give up. Hey, I hope you switch overnight! But most can't do that. What I found out is that your body and mind are addicted to the chemicals you taste in whole milk.

You think you like that momentary pleasure. So you have to deal with what's going on in your mind. This is true about any and every food you are addicted to. IF you crave it or make excuses for not switching to a healthier version of a product, then you are addicted to that product. I hear that about milk only second to soda pops.

Lactose intolerance keeps some people from drinking milk. But because doctors have no cures and deliberately refuse to tell you any solution to any health problem, the cure for lactose intolerance is never used by doctors. But there is a cure for lactose intolerance. Lactose intolerance occurs when your small intestine doesn't make enough of the enzyme called lactase. Lactase breaks down the natural sugar in milk called lactose. So without enough lactase to digest the lactose in milk, that lactose remains undigested in your intestinal tract causing gas, bloating, pain and cramps in the lower belly.

What doctors call lactose intolerance is the result of your body becoming acidic by habitually consuming sugars, animal products, white flour and chlorinated water. Chlorinated water also destroys the beneficial bacteria that are necessary to digest food and maintain a healthy immune system. The result is an acidic body in which thousands of body metabolisms no longer occur, like not producing enough lactase to prevent lactose intolerance.

With your acidic body not being able to digest the natural sugar in milk, called lactose, it sits in your intestines "boiling" in its acidic environment. This is what causes all the symptoms of lactose intolerance. But as you can now understand, no one is really lactose intolerant. You are lactose intolerant only because your body is acidic AND you have a Magnesium deficiency.

To cure yourself, drink ½ teaspoon baking soda (sodium bicarbonate) in 6 ounces of filtered water 3 to 5 times daily and take at least 250mg to 400mg Magnesium 3-4 times daily. Do this for at least 6-8 weeks, then every other day or so. Do this while you clean up your diet and drinks to start eliminating as much sugars, high fructose corn syrup, animal products and chlorinated water as possible.

But even once you end your doctor named "lactose intolerance", if you don't avoid the saturation of poisons in your diet and take Magnesium oxide supplements regularly, your lactose intolerance will return; just as science dictates that it will.

Once again you see how two of the things used to cure all disease can cure your lactose intolerance – Magnesium and baking soda.

You now have filtered water, black tea (Lipton) sweetened with Stevia, Brown Pure Cane Sugar, several fruit juices and 2% and Skim milk that you can drink. But you can also drink some herbal teas. When we have herbal tea at our house, we make 2 cups at a time; one each for my wife and I.

The most medicinal herbs are Lemon Balm and Sage. Both are "cure alls". Lemon Balm was a cure for everything with the Egyptians, while Sage is a "cure all" for Native American Indians.

To make any tea from fresh or dried herbs, take 2 teaspoons of dried herb for each cup, 8-ounces, of water. Or use fresh herbs that you believe would equal 2 teaspoons dry. Place the herbs in each cup. Boil your filtered water and pour over the herbs. Let steep for 5 minutes. Then add a teaspoon or two of raw honey or Brown pure cane sugar.

Do not be limited by the few herbs I mention. All herbs are natural plant medicines. And although Sage and Lemon Balm are "cure alls", there are many useful herbs. Some worth mentioning are Chamomile, Hawthorn Berries, Valerian Root, Cinnamon, Garlic, Astragalus, Alisma, Peppermint, Echinacea, Rosemary, Ginger root, Turmeric, Basil, Butcher's Broom, Black Cohosh, Eyebright, Maca root, St. John's Wort, Stevia and Saw Palmetto. And there are so many more not named.

Most can be bought as spices, while others come in pill form and others can be grown. There are only specific ones that are commonly drank as a tea. Those are Chamomile, Rosemary, Basil, Cinnamon and Stevia. But you can also find almost any herb in tea bags, ready to steep and drink. So you can spend a lot of time having fun enjoying many herbal teas that not only taste good, but present a near endless array of tastes and benefits.

Bottled Water

What about bottled water? The simple answer is...don't be a fool! Buying bottled water is foolish and a waste of money, unless there are some odd circumstances I haven't thought of. If the gas company has fracked your water supply you could need bottled water. Fracked water will ruin your water filter in no time!

Bottled water contains more than water. I looked and looked and looked for bottled WATER, but could only find bottled water with several other ingredients! The best bottled water I found was Ozarka. It has the fewest ingredients. You can get hundreds of times as much pure filtered water for your money by buying a counter-top fluoride water filter than you get buying bottled water by the case.

Bottled water is just tap water in a bottle. But fluoride filtered water is pure. Bottled water never is. So your body has to filter out those added ingredients. I bought bottled water one time, and that was enough to convince me to never buy any more.

If bottled water didn't have chlorine in it, there would be bacteria growing in it after a few weeks. You won't see chlorine in the ingredients because the chlorine is already in the tap water. So you only have to list "water" as an ingredient, even though it contains chlorine and fluoride.

As you can see, bottled water is not a healthy choice. Your money is best spent on a high quality water filter such as a multi-stage fluoride filter; or invest in an Osmosis system for all the water in your home. But even a carbon water filter will remove at least 90% of the chlorine; faucet-end filters, counter-top and pitcher filters.

I would also advise you to avoid alkaline waters, for many reasons. The claims the makers of these make are mostly hype. One even claims to have the best water on the planet, better than God's water! You are far better off with a multi-stage fluoride filter and baking soda water to make your pure water alkaline whenever you choose; and for a whole lot less!

Poisons In Your Food

You could write a huge book just pointing out all the chemicals in our food supply and the details of how harmful all of them are. The excuses for putting all these chemicals in our food do not, and never could, justify this saturation of poisons; not to mention that most of the poisons in your food are put there to addict you to their products. Drugging people is illegal, but there is no government to enforce any of these laws.

There is even a law in at least one State that states that anyone who makes or sells drugs that are the direct cause of anyone's death has committed a felony. But no matter how many people are killed by these drugs in our food, and drinks, no corporation has been prosecuted for those crimes. Same is true with the 25,000-100,000 Americans that prescription drugs kill every year. No doctor or drug corporation has been prosecuted for any of the millions of deaths directly caused by THEIR drugs.

So the only chance for you to avoid being killed by food corporations, drug corporations and doctors, is to recognize their deadly drugs and avoid them. But since all drugs are certified "safe" by the FDA, corporations are free to drug you and addict you to their drugs regardless of how many people their drugs kill each and every year. And unless you learn what I am about to tell you, and practice it, the only way you won't die from these drugs is IF you die of an accident before their drugs kill you.

It's a fact that 90% of Americans die of disease. And out of that 90%, it's estimated that as much as 95% of those people die from the food they eat.

Our food supplies are saturated with all kinds of poisons. But the most used and abused poisons are never called the drugs and poisons that they ARE! Those two drugs are white granulated sugar and white flour. Reducing and eliminating these two common drug foods from your diet will be the most drastic improvement most of you can make in pursuit of a healthy diet.

And when you are looking for healthy products to buy, you get tricked into buying a product that is almost always worse for you, with false and tricky labeling. That includes the misleading terms "All Natural", "Low Salt", "Low Calorie", "Low Fat" and "Diet"; as well as the terms "From Concentrate" and "100% Juice" on fruit juice labels.

Reading labels must be a way of life with you if you are going to clean up your current diet. If your current diet and lifestyle is just fine, you wouldn't be sick. So I am telling you how and why to change that for yourself.

YOU made you sick. And it is YOU that can cure yourself.

I am teaching you about the sciences you used to make yourself sick. But I am mostly teaching you about the sciences that heal your body.

It is YOUR BODY that heals itself. So as silly as it sounds, anyone with a BODY can cure themselves using natural science.

And for those who doubt what I just said, let me ask you this. Have you ever cut yourself? Do you still have that cut? Oh, so your body healed itself, right? Well of course your body healed itself.

So we use science, the Laws of Physics, to make our body do what we want it to do; which is heal itself. You already know to get water filters, take Magnesium, Vitamin C and Fish oil. But the reason you have to start every cure by drinking baking soda water is that your body has become acidic from the habitual consumption of sugars, white flour, meats and other animal products, as well as chlorinated water.

So short of telling you the only way you will ever cure yourself is IF you become a vegetarian, I am including all the following information to help you clean up your current diet as much as possible.

A major point of this book is to keep things as short and simple as possible. So the information is not complete, but enough to get your diet cleaned up real well. It's not that hard to do either.

We covered the facts about sugars and sweeteners back when I was telling you to watch what you drink. So you need to reference those facts when trying to clean up the sugars in your food too.

You also have to remember that high fructose corn syrup is in everything you eat and drink! No matter how it does NOT belong in a product, it most likely is in that product anyway. It HAS to be. High fructose is THE drug that addicts you to a product. So it's always in there. It's in most bread too.

You have to try and avoid all products that list high fructose corn syrup in the ingredients. And if it's listed in the first 4 ingredients, it should be on your red alert list to avoid altogether.

The front line in the battle to clean up your diet is at the grocery store. It's at the grocery store where you get almost all your food. So that's where your efforts have to begin in order to clean up your current diet.

Read labels – Merely reading the manufacturer's label is usually enough information for you to know to avoid a product. Read labels in the grocery store and at home. Reading labels at the grocery store keeps a lot of bad products out of your grocery cart. So they never make it out the door with you and into your home.

And whatever products you bring home, you should be reading the labels to back up your efforts at the grocery store. A lot of times you can't read the ingredients because the letters are so tiny or blend with the color of the label.

Also, a lot of products that don't have high fructose corn syrup at one time, will soon be found in that same product later on. And even products that say No High Fructose Corn Syrup, soon do. A good example of that is Hunt's "No HFCS" ketchup. We haven't been able to find it since early 2013.

Low salt, Low Fat, Low Calorie? These are the most common terms used by corporations to trick you into thinking you are buying a healthy product. If a product contains all 3 of these, it will be low in one and higher in the other 2 than in the regular version of the item. If it's labeled "Low fat", it will be lower in fat but higher in salt and sugar than the regular version.

The higher in fat, sugar and salt a product is, the greater the sensation it gives your body. But food is for nourishing the body! And the damage these poisons do to your body is what helps to develop "disease" in your body.

So read the labels to confirm these facts. The simple solution is to stick with the regular versions of products instead of being seduced into believing that products labeled "Low fat", "Low Salt" and "Low Calorie" are somehow good for you; and worth the higher prices.

I explained about sugars earlier. The same sugars found in most drinks, saturate a great portion of our food supplies. The most common one-two punch of poisons in our food supply is white flour and sugar. This is what makes up the content of most cookies, cakes, cereals and even breads.

Bread – Whole wheat or white?

Since the wheat germ and wheat bran are removed from wheat to create what is known as "white flour", the answer is easily Whole wheat.

Even when you buy bread that says it is whole wheat bread, it rarely is. They use the term whole wheat and state on the label that it is wheat flour, enriched wheat flour. Whole wheat is stated as "whole wheat flour" or "Stone ground whole wheat flour". And, of course, this is not isolated to just bread.

Although whole wheat buns, rolls and other pastries are hard to find, the same is true with all of them. Finding whole wheat items in restaurants is even more rare than in the grocery stores.

The best solution is to learn to make cookies, cakes, cobblers, cinnamon rolls, dinner rolls and others with whole wheat flour. You can also substitute whole wheat flour for white flour in recipes, just as you substitute brown pure cane sugar for white granulated sugar in recipes.

It is your body that dictates the fact that white flour is almost pure poison, by removing almost all of the white flour you eat! So take the time to avoid white flour. I have eaten whole wheat and other whole grain breads since 1981. I have only eaten white bread on occasions, but never regularly.

We try to stick with a generic brand whole wheat bread like Best Choice, but also eat Nature's Own Whole Wheat bread and 100% Whole Grain bread.

Making your own breads and doughs for most items that require white flour, is another thing we do to keep from being forced to consume white flour. Failing to do so will cause your intestines to bleed and more.

What about meat – red meat, pork, chicken, turkey, fish?

The best solution is to avoid meat altogether. Eat fish, fish types that have scales. Most classify fish as meat. But I classify it as fish, since meat comes from animals with blood. I prefer to use the classifications red meat, fish and fowl. This clarifies the level of poisons in what meat you eat. Red meat has the most. Then Pork. Chicken is third. Turkey is fourth. And fish are the least poisonous and also the most beneficial of all meats.

All red meat and pork are the dead cut up parts of cows and pigs. We eat it without ever calling it "dead cow flesh" or "dead pig flesh". It's bad enough that they are slaughtered in inhumane ways. But add to that all the antibiotics, growth hormones and other drugs they are injected with, and you have poison-saturated meat. Not to mention that they feed on poison-saturated feed and in many cases, live in unsanitary conditions.

Pigs eat their own feces and also wallow in it. But we don't like to think about these things. So we blindly poison ourselves by eating too much of what we should really only be eating none or very little of. The so-called "American diet" consists of red meat and sugar; which is the diet of a savage. It has created the greatest plague of disease that any nation has ever had. Not even the Bubonic plague was more devastating than your dear "American diet". Nope, the Bubonic plague only had 50 Million victims.

But the US has at least 150 Million people that are permanently sick. And the rest of the country is sick most of the time. I use to think I was never sick. But that's because headaches and heartburn didn't count. I ate white flour, sugar, red meat, other meats and never thought about it as a kid or teenager.

But by continuing your habitual "American diet" the only result anyone is getting from it is one chronic disease after another. So that is why I went into some details about the devastation red meat and sugar have done to the health of our entire nation. To continue to believe you can have different results from this same behavior is not rational or possible.

While you are working on your addiction to red meat, with all the fat and drugs in it, you can still eat fish, turkey, chicken, some pork and some ground Chuck on occasion.

Fish is the most expensive. Tuna is about $1 per canned 5-ounces. Salmon is about $3 a pound in the can. Fresh or frozen fish is at least $5-$8 a pound. So eating chicken at 1/3 the price is something most of us have to do. I don't think it's reasonable to expect you to spend 4 or 5 times as much on your groceries in order to cure yourself. And the safest choices for meat are quite costly, while chicken is the most cost efficient choice meat choice.

Pond raised fish are usually saturated with all the chemicals that are put in the water they are raised in. And with fish without scales, like catfish, these chemicals soak into the bodies of the fish very easily. Talapia, Cod and Salmon are excellent fish choices, as well as Tuna. But use those canned with water instead of oil. Draining either will help a lot.

Buying ground beef is about as risky as you can get when buying meat. Most of it is acceptable. But there are large amounts of ground beef that are mixed with the ground parts of animals and other substances that are a cause for alarm. Here's what Wikipedia states about this "pink slime" that is added to a large quantity of our ground beef supply:

It (pink slime) is produced by processing low-grade beef trimmings and other meat by-products such as cartilage, connective tissue and sinew which contain fat and small amounts of lean beef, and mechanically separating the lean beef from the fat through the use of a centrifuge at about 100°F (38°C).

The heat liquefies the fat to help separate lean beef from fat and other by-products. The recovered beef material is processed, heated, and treated with gaseous ammonia or citric acid to kill E. coli, salmonella, and other bacteria. Gaseous ammonia in contact with the water in the meat produces ammonium hydroxide. The product is finely ground, compressed into pellets or blocks, flash frozen and then shipped for use as an additive.

The more fat in the meat, the more chemicals the meat contains; since chemicals tend to accumulate in body fat. It's the fat in meat that causes your veins and arteries to clog. And when you add vegetable oils inside your body, scarred and clogged veins and arteries are sure to come.

Taking fish oil will delay that a while. But when your problem is all the fat and oils you consume, the solution is to reduce the amount of fat and oils you consume. So cut back on the red meat and pork. Eat more fish, chicken and turkey. And cut back on the oils you consume. That's why the next thing you need to learn about are oils.

Oils – Vegetable, Olive, Canola, Coconut?

You all choke down gobs and gobs of vegetable oils. It's bad enough that you cook in vegetable oil. But most of the vegetable oil you consume doesn't come from the foods soaked in vegetable oil that you fry at home. The biggest source of vegetable oils is in processed foods like Oreo cookies, Twinkies, potato chips, breads, cakes, pies, peanut butter and margarine! I'm not picking on just these food products. The grocery store shelves are packed with vegetable oil saturated food products like the ones I just named. You need to look for trans-fat content on the label and avoid any products that have any trans-fats in the ingredients. Look for partially hydrogenated oils. Trans-fats are a byproduct created during partial dehydrogenation.

But beware! Just because the label lists trans-fats as zero, they can still have trans fats. Food manufacturers only list trans fats above zero if the product contains at least 0.5 grams of trans-fats per serving. They even fix the labeling per serving many times so they can claim their products contain zero trans-fats on the label. Trans-fats reduce the amount of good, HDL, cholesterol in your body. So if the ingredients list partially dehydrogenated oil of any kind, avoid that product. Do not buy it. But no matter how well you solve this problem in your home, you still scarf down good amounts of vegetable oils when you eat any restaurant food.

There is no need to single out any one restaurant or many restaurants! Your whole problem with eating restaurant food is that none of it is healthy. They'll put out a salad bar at some places instead of cooking in Canola oil, using whole wheat flour, raw honey and no high fructose corn syrup. They are in business to make money and make as much money as they can within the Laws of this country. The problem is how we don't have a real government in this country any more. So it doesn't matter how bad these substances in the food supply are, as long as it's FDA approved.

All the fried food you eat in restaurants is cooked in vegetable oils. The damage those oils do to your body creates that craving for all the poison soaked foods and drinks you consume. It's that added taste that vegetable oils give foods that are cooked in vegetable oils. You think that chicken is good for you from that famous fried chicken restaurant, even though it's soaked in those artery clogging vegetable oils.

About the only thing you can do about this is stop eating restaurant food; especially the big chain franchise restaurants. I have known of a smaller local restaurant that cooked in Canola oil and offered Whole wheat bread as an option for their sandwiches. Eating restaurant food is a serious health risk for you and your family. So don't let anyone distract you from your choice to avoid consuming foods and drinks that are bad for your health.

The only restaurant whose food I eat is almost always SubWay. I always get my sandwiches on multi-grain bread. SubWay is the healthiest restaurant eating I know of. We cut out our eating out by about 80%; from most days to maybe once every 2 to 3 months.

But hey, since eating out costs at least twice as much and is twice as poisonous as the same food if you cook it at home, you've convinced yourself that you are "living the good life". When the fact is, that there is very little chance of eating anything healthy from 99% of the restaurants. Eating at home is the all-around best idea for sure.

Eating at home is always going to be more healthy and cheaper than any food you can get in restaurants; especially the well-known fast food chains. And you don't have to worry about how filthy their kitchen is or about any of their employees spitting in your food or tainting it in other ways.

Olive oil is the best oil to use by far. Extra virgin olive oil is the best olive oil. Virgin olive oil is almost as good a quality as Extra Virgin Olive oil, but is not. I always buy Extra Virgin Olive oil for about $6 a quart. My wife uses olive oil to oil the skillet to cook grilled sandwiches and other light oiling cooking jobs. You can also whip up some mayonnaise using olive oil. It will last about 2 weeks in the refrigerator. Olive oil has many health benefits and has some great health care uses I bet most of you are unaware of! Always keep some olive oil in your home, and use it efficiently to make it go a long way. If money is no object, use it generously. The more you use olive oil, the better your health is going to be.

Use Olive oil on your hair. Cover your hair with Olive oil. Let it sit all night. Shampoo your hair the next morning and see how soft your hair is! It's also good on burns and any dry skin you may have.

The best all-around oil is Canola oil. Although it doesn't have the extensive health benefits that olive oil has, Canola oil is about 25% the cost of Extra Virgin Olive Oil. Canola oil costs the same as vegetable oils. With that fact in mind, I can't understand why anyone would buy vegetable oil instead of Canola oil! There is no known damage which Canola oil does to your body. On the contrary! There are lots of people who take a tablespoon or two of Canola oil for their hearts most days.

Canola oil has the lowest saturated fat content of all oils; including olive oil. It is very high in unsaturated fats too. Because of Canola oil's excellent health benefits, I suggest you read more about Canola oil and olive oil, and SEARCH the INTERNET too.

You do have to be careful when buying Canola oil, since 80% of the Canola oil made in this country is a GMO, Genetically Modified Organism. This is not true about Canola oil from outside the US, like Canada and Europe. Canola is really Canadian Low Acid Oil. Use expeller-pressed, non-GMO canola oil. I use very little oil for anything. So none of this is much of a concern to me. Just remember that almost all vegetable oils are GMO too. So Canola oil is still the better choice.

Coconut oil is the best choice for high heat cooking. But finding it is the problem most of us face. You can't use something you can't get. So I have to keep that in mind when telling you about oils.

Coconut oil, which is an edible oil that is extracted from the meat of coconuts, has the most health benefits of any oil. You can even cook with it at high heat and not destroy the beneficial substances in the oil. No other oil can do this at high heat. Coconut oil doesn't begin being destroyed, burnt up, until it reaches 351 degrees Fahrenheit.

Also, peanut oil has the most (good) mono unsaturated fat, other than olive and Canola oil. Sunflower oil is also a better choice than vegetable oils, but still lags behind olive, Canola and peanut oil as far as overall health benefits. But it's still a much better choice than artery clogging vegetable oils. So avoid using vegetable oils by making the healthier choice at the grocery store. Stock up on it when it's on sale.

Eggs

The USDA classifies eggs as meat due to their high protein content. Just because some eggs are brown doesn't mean they are healthier than white eggs. You have to make sure those brown eggs are actually organic eggs. To comply with USDA requirements to be able to label eggs as organic, the eggs have to come from chickens that have been fed organic feed and are free of antibiotics; as well as better standards for the welfare of the chickens.

The way to tell the difference between poison eggs and eggs that are mostly free of poisons, is by the taste. The best eggs are Organic eggs. Organic eggs don't have that chemical bite that regular eggs do. You will begin to recognize that chemical bite in regular eggs after you've eaten organic eggs a few times. You can also cook Organic and regular eggs and taste them both, side by side, to easily tell.

It's this chemical bite or burn you should focus on while eating eggs, or anything, in order to recognize how poisonous or healthy any food item is.

A good choice for eggs is Eggland Eggs. Eggland Eggs are organic eggs. These eggs come from chickens that are fed an organic vegetarian diet.

But even if you just eat regular non-Organic eggs, eggs are good for you; especially if you compare the nutritional value of eggs to red meat or some sugary cereal. And a couple of large eggs only costs about 35 cents!

Eggs are one of the most nutritious foods there is. A large egg is about 77 calories, 6 grams protein, 5 grams of healthy fats and provide good amounts of Vitamins A, B5, B12, B2, Folate and Phosphorous. A large egg also provides about 1/4 of your daily need for Selenium. Eggs also contain decent amounts of Zinc, Calcium and Vitamins B6, D, E and K. Eggs also contain good amounts of Choline; which flushes fat out of your liver.

Although eggs contain high amounts of cholesterol, they do not raise your cholesterol levels in the blood. Your liver will produce less cholesterol when you eat eggs. Only people with certain genetic disorders should avoid eggs. If you think you are allergic to eggs, try Organic eggs. You most likely can't tolerate the poisons in regular eggs. It's those chemicals in those eggs that are causing the "allergic" reaction. Simply put, you are most likely having a chemical reaction, not an allergic reaction.

You should also always be aware of the fact that when your body is acidic, you get all kinds of diseases. As your body becomes more and more acidic, the more likely it is for any chemicals to cause a quick, undesirable reaction. This factual science applies to things like lactose intolerance all the way to food allergies. Once your acidic body ceases to be able to perform more and more metabolisms, even eating nuts or grains will make you sick.

But the first problem you solve is the acidic state of your body. Once that is done you won't have bad reactions to common foods. And although eggs are classified as meat and are indeed animal products, eggs still come from a bird, contain no blood and add nothing bad to your body. You only get a small amount of poisons from eating regular eggs, and even a smaller amount with Organic eggs.

And at $2 a large dozen, I can only speak in favor of eating plenty of eggs.

Once you've learned to avoid all the chemical sugars, white flour, high fructose corn syrup, red meat and vegetable oils, you are more than well on your way to a much healthier life and body. You are ridding your body of all disease by restoring it to health Naturally.

I am trying to make the point that regardless of what name or names that doctors have given to the accumulations of poisons in your body and the bad effects of your chronic diet deficiencies, you restore your body to health to rid your body of all those diseases.

Every time you think about eating or drinking something, think about this – Do I want to eat something that will help my body to repair damaged cells

OR do I want to eat or drink something my body will work hours to remove from my body after it damages me internally first?

The more you choose to eat and drink something that will build your body, the faster you move toward complete healing of all disease. While every choice to eat or drink something you know is saturated with poisons, takes you backwards into your diseases.

To help you even further, I am adding the next chapter to tell you other things you can do to speed your healing along. Although you already know the most important things to do, lets go ahead and learn what else helps.

I'll start off by telling you what you can do about the soaps, shampoos, lotions, deodorants and other personal hygiene items. They're all saturated with chemicals or are just nothing BUT chemicals.

So here's what I know about that...............

5 - Other Things That Help

There are other things you can do that help you restore your body to health. We have covered the major things. All of those have a direct impact on the health of your body. But other things like your attitude, reading labels, fasting, exercise and even your attitude at the grocery store can all help get you cured of all diseases.

I mentioned attitude and your attitude at the grocery store separately. Your attitude is about cures. Cures are not a part of the modern medical profession. So you would have to learn about cures from someone besides doctors. This alone is enough to confuse you. Doctors are suppose to cure, heal, you. But because they make many times more money treating your diseases, that is what they do. And you are left without cures.

See, we are blind to this self-evident reality that doctors cure no one; even though it is reality for all of us. It's cures that don't have a place anywhere. So you have to make places for cures; for the restoration of your body to health to end all disease. This seems like a bad thing, but it's not.

You can cure yourself of all diseases and never have to suffer any disease again; not even headaches! And all of it is Natural and doesn't include big sums of money being paid to doctors. So without doctors involved your cost of everything goes down at least 90%. You get cured for about a penny on the dollar. for what you would pay a doctor to treat you just one time.

Attitude - Your attitude about this will have an impact on whether you get cured and how long it will take to realize it. Everyone is told by their doctors that there is no cure for the diseases they have. And that's the end of it. Your god has spoken and his word is final. So you don't even look for a cure. And your life is over because this leaves you with no hope.

I get attacked by the medical profession in some book reviews at Amazon. And they all insist there is no cure for kidney disease or any disease. Some suggest you check with the Mayo Clinic or take the word of the doctors they work for, who refuse to cure anyone. But all there is to say about that is "Yes that is exactly what I point out. Doctors cure no one.

But I cured myself of 11 diseases doctors call "chronic" because they REFUSE to cure anyone. They are misleading people because they fear they will be punished for being a part of the most incompetent profession our nation has ever known. 150,000,000 Americans with at least one chronic, permanent, disease, is the proof of this self-evident fact.

Everything I say in my books is to set YOU, the Individual, free of disease and the Death it brings for 90% of Americans. Your attitude is the big boy that rules over your mind. And if you don't seek a cure, there is no possibility of you ever finding cures. Seek cures and you will find them.

I am reminded of a man whose daughter was dying of cancer and was told there's no cure. She was sure to die before long. But this man sought a cure and found it. It wasn't the cure for all disease I am telling you. It wasn't even the cure for cancer 17-year old Angela Zhang discovered either. There are cures for all disease. But if you want to be rid of all diseases and maintain that freedom from disease, you are going to have to know all the things I have told you so far in this book; regardless of where you learn all of this.

Your attitude in the grocery store is just that, the attitude you have at the grocery store and about choosing the things on your grocery list. What you need to do is develop the attitude that you buy what you know is best for you and your family. Spend time in the grocery store reading labels. And have a chip on your shoulder toward the vast array of poison-saturated items that fill at least 80% of all grocery store shelves.

Just refusing to buy any items with high fructose corn syrup in them will eliminate about 2/3 of the items in grocery stores! So most people buy bad foods because it takes some information to avoid doing so. The more you read labels, the better you will be at avoiding poisons in your food and drinks.

By reading labels, you will find out that there aren't any choices when it comes to mayonnaise, ketchup, Bar-B-Q sauce, most salad dressings and other condiments. Poisons are as much as half the contents of those products. And finding one that isn't, is next to impossible to do.

There is no ketchup without high fructose corn syrup. Two kinds of Bar-B-Q Sauces, one type mayonnaise and the rest of your condiments are almost as bad. The 2 best kinds of Bar-B-Q sauce are Garland Jack Secret X and Wickers. Wickers is $3.79 for an 18-ounce bottle and Garland Jack is almost $3. The cheap ones like Kraft are packed with high fructose corn syrup.

The only mayonnaise we use is Kraft's Mayonnaise. It only has sugar. That makes it the better choice over all the high fructose corn syrup packed ones; which is pretty much all the rest.

If you want salad dressing, you will have to use the ones like Ranch and oil dressings to avoid all the high fructose corn syrup. So reading labels when you are in the grocery store will give you all the information you need to avoid the saturation of poisons in all our food and drinks.

Your attitude about grocery shopping in and out of the grocery store is your front line of defense in guarding you and your family from all these poisons. If you never put them in your grocery cart, you can't bring them home. And that's the attitude you need to have and live by.

Exercise – Although I don't know of any diseases caused by lack of exercise, I do realize what benefits it can have in speeding your healing along. It does strengthen your heart, which is beneficial. But the thing exercise does that helps cure you is that it pumps oxygen into your body.

This is important because all diseased cells are low in oxygen. Cancer cells have about 1/3 less oxygen as healthy cells. The more acidic your body, the less oxygen cells will have. Of course, the thing you do for that is drink baking soda water. But the more oxygen you can pump into your body, the healthier cells will be.

But because people die from exercise, I don't push exercise as something you must do to cure yourself. But exercise is needed to restore your body to health. Inactivity tends to lead to a better chance of getting sick. So exercise in moderation. Stick with low impact exercise until exercise is a habit. And get as much of your exercise doing useful activities as you can. Running on a treadmill, lifting weights and all the types of exercises you can do are not what I could ever recommend.

The US puts a huge reward on exercising. But yet doesn't dare mention cures or anything that can cure you. The rewards of exercising 20 minutes a day for 3 or 4 days a week for a year only pale in comparison to the rewards of avoiding poisons. Even drinking pure filtered water is too; as well as drinking baking soda water or correcting your major diet deficiencies. The rewards of doing so can't be bought no matter how much money you have!

So put these things in perspective and don't end up sick because you thought regular exercise would keep disease away! Two other things that do you more good than exercise are fasting and doing something about all the chemicals that make up most of your personal hygiene items like soap, shampoo, lotion, toothpaste, deodorant, make up and more.

Fasting – Fasting forces your body to use its energy to repair damaged cells and remove toxins. Freeing up the energy used for digesting so that all that energy can be used to heal your body, is one of the most useful things you can do to cure yourself. But since people usually don't have the willpower to fast, I can't place too much emphasis on fasting; although if you do fast, the results will be quite beneficial.

There is no need to fast for days or weeks at a time. You can do as many 16 hour fasts as you want. A 16 hour fast, as I call it, would be done by eating your last meal about 6 or 7 pm. Then not eating again until about 10 in the morning or noon. You would drink cold pure filtered water to douse the hunger pains. You can also drink some pure juice from almost any produce. You would need a juicer to do that effectively.

Drinking a sugary drink, like some store-bought Orange juice, will only make you feel hungrier. Same with most any food; although you can always eat a slice of Apple, Orange or other fruit to help hold down your urges to eat a bunch of food. Same is true if you drink baking soda water or take probiotics. When the bad bacteria in your stomach is well out-numbered by the good bacteria, you get hungry again about 90 minutes after you eat.

You need 80% good bacteria and 20% bad bacteria to have a normal healthy stomach and intestinal tract. But because you drank chlorinated water for years, that chlorine has kept killing the bacteria inside you too. And combine that with all the acidic things we consume, our stomachs and intestinal tracts are barren. It's this barren state that causes you to feel hungry in as little as an hour and an half after eating a good meal.

You should continue taking Magnesium, Vitamin C and Fish oil when you are fasting. So resort to food only after you have taken these as usual, drank the baking soda water and drank pure water, but still need something to stop the hunger pains and stomach growling.

And remember to refrain from fasting for days if your sickness makes you feel bad. You need to do all the other things to get your body healing itself before your body is strong enough to do without food. Fast for 16 hours as often as you can. There are numerous things that can detox the body to one degree or another. But fasting while drinking pure filtered water is the best detox of all. I can't emphasis this enough!!!

You can stretch your fasts beyond 16 hours when you know you are safe in doing so. The practice of Hippocrates, the father of medicine, was based on fasting and herbs. So although fasting is as irrelevant to doctors as cures are, it is a powerful exercise in forcing your body to heal itself.

Another important thing you need to do is, clean up the poisons in your personal hygiene items and related products. Here's some help to do that.

Personal hygiene items – soaps, shampoos, lotions, make up, toothpaste, deodorants and more. All of these items are poison-saturated, unless you know what to look for.

Every soap and shampoo you can get is just about all chemicals. So looking for any soap or shampoo that isn't so bad for you is another hard task. But once you find out where you can get soaps that are natural, you will be glad you aren't soaking yourself with more chemicals just by using soap.

You can buy Dr. Bonner's soaps and shampoos. Although their bars of soap are 3 or 4 times higher than chemical soaps, it lasts about 3 times as long as the chemical soaps. So the cost is not really that much higher to use a safer, natural soap. You can also use the soap to wash your hair. But they also have safe, Organic shampoos.

Other soaps like Seaweed soap, Olive oil soaps and Glycerin soaps are all good natural soaps and can be purchased at Puritan's. Tea tree oil is another good choice for natural soap.

The best toothpaste I know of is plain ole baking soda. Just wet your brush under running water and dip it bristles down in a box of baking soda. Brush all over your teeth and squish it around in your mouth. This will neutralize the acid on your teeth and gums and make them fell squeaky clean. Doing this before bed time gives you a whole eight hours with no acid eating your gums and enamel on your teeth.

You can also use dry baking soda as a deodorant. It works as good or better than any chemical deodorant. The only problem you will have is from your body being too acidic. If this is the case, you will get reddening of your underarms that tends to burn and sting. This is from the alkaline baking soda neutralizing all the acid in your sweat.

Just barely dampen a fingertip or two. Dip them in the box of baking soda and rub on your underarms. You can also use a small brush like a make up brush to apply it to your underarms. And I didn't mention all the money you will save from now on by using baking soda as your toothpaste and/or as your deodorant. All natural and even better than their chemical counterparts.

And in case you are wondering about the current deodorant you are using! Those aluminum compounds in your underarm deodorants are causing those knots, lumps, under your arms. Aluminium chloride, aluminum chlorohydrate, and aluminum-zirconium compounds, most notably aluminum zirconium tetrachlorohydrex gly and aluminum zirconium trichlorohydrex gly, are frequently used in antiperspirants.

Aluminium chlorohydrate and aluminum zirconium tetrachlorohydrate gly are the most frequent active ingredients in commercial antiperspirants. So if you have lumps or knots in your arm pits, stop using that deodorant with an aluminum based ingredient. Those knots are from you poisoning your lymph nodes so excessively that they are swollen. It's that simple.

Using these chemical deodorants takes a toll on your lymph nodes, which is critical because your lymph system is the backup, reinforcement, of your body's immune system. So this daily poisoning needs to end.

Over-the-counter medications are also pure poison. You can use natural substitutes for most of them. But once you are doing things like drinking baking soda water, taking Vitamin C, Magnesium and Fish oil, you won't be needing the chemical ant-acids or the aspirin, Aleve, Tylenol or Ibuprofen. Your headaches and heartburn will fade away.

Any heartburn should be dealt with by drinking baking soda water when you get heartburn. Taking TUMS is pretty effective since TUMS is mostly Calcium carbonate. I noticed sucrose is now the main ingredient though. The pH of Calcium carbonate is 9.4, compared to baking soda at pH 8.5.

Your cold and flu remedy should be to do the same thing. Taking 1000mg Vitamin C every 3-4 hours while you have a cold or flu will bring it to an end in 2-3 days. Taking Astragalus, Echinacea and/or monolaurin are all a big help. Dry Cinnamon mixed in a few ounces of applesauce will soothe and heal that scratchy throat and coughing. And of course, drinking Apple Cider vinegar will help bring you out of a cold or flu.

So why scarf down all those chemical cough medicines, cold medicines, throat lozenges and throat sprays, when you can use Natural things to heal your body and not hurt it. What little help you get from the chemicals is negated by the fact your body has to use its energy to remove ALL those chemical medicines.

That dental pain can also be handled pretty well naturally. You should rinse your teeth and gums with warm baking soda water. Sea salt water is a good second choice. If the pain persists, use a Q-tip to put Cinnamon oil or Clove oil on the painful area. It actually works real well. It will blister your gums if you overuse it. This is a great thing to do when your dentist tells you they can give you an appointment for days or weeks!

Baking soda, Cinnamon oil and Clove oil to the rescue for your dental problems. You also need to clean up your lotions and makeup.

Lotions and makeup – are rubbed on your skin and seep into your pores. If you're using a shower filter, you won't have a need for any lotions. Instead of using lotions on dry skin or dandruff shampoos, get a shower filter. If your skin, hair or scalp get dry, just rub Olive oil on them. No chemicals. All good!

Makeup is mostly chemicals. On average there are about 26 chemicals in eye shadow, 33 in lipstick and an average of 16 in blush. By comparison, shampoo and deodorant has about 15, body lotion has 32 and fake tan products average about 22 chemicals in those products.

I'm not a woman. So I don't know what you can substitute for any of your toxic makeup items. My wife just does without makeup except for certain special occasions. Give your face and skin some breaks from makeup.

If you want more detailed information about specific things you can do for all kinds of ailments and diseases, get my book Natural Healing – BOOK of CURES. It gives you more vitamins, herbs and other natural substances you can take to help target specific diseases to cure them more quickly.

It also gives you ways to deal with back pain and bee stings, along with other beneficial things you can do to end your cancer, heart disease, erectile dysfunction, arthritis, kidney disease and more.

What this book is for is to give you the most important information you need to restore your body to health to rid your body of all diseases. And do so in as few words and pages as possible.

So I left out all the long-winded explanations of things and just told you what to do to cure yourself. I also made it clear that what we are really doing is restoring your body to health. And once you do that, you no longer have any diseases. **I am at the end of talking about diseases! Teaching you how to heal your body and keep it healthy makes disease a moot issue.**

My Final Words

The idea of this book was to give you the best information available to get you cured of all disease and do so in the fewest words I could. Anyone who is dying of chronic disease needs help and needs it quickly. So every minute you spend reading had to count. That is the major reason behind this book.

The other major reason I wrote this book was to state the transition from saying we are curing disease, to seeing all of this as merely restoring your body to health. If you had known how to take care of your body in the first place, you wouldn't have gotten sick at all.

But you think you can eat, drink and use anything you choose, without any consequences. But that is not true. You can't beat science and its Laws of Physics. So you end up dying of disease just as 90% of all Americans do.

First you get sick, mainly from corporations deliberately addicting you to the drugs they saturated our food and drinks with. Then doctors and their medical profession finish you off with all their treatments, tests, chemical medicines and medical procedures; but never cure you.

Change for the better with doctors and their medical profession is never going to happen. There are no cures in the medical profession because money is their reason for existing; not the health of people. So you can either wait on your beloved doctors to start curing people as they are suppose to do, OR you can empower yourself with the knowledge to cure yourself and maintain that health for the rest of your life. The choice is always yours.

For those who choose Life over Death, good health over disease, well-being over suffering, no pain over pain and reality over perversion, are the ones who are listening to this.

Even if I was a total liar, the fact that you have no cures and refuse to listen to anyone who tells you there ARE cures, is only proving that YOU have no desire to be cured or be healthy! Seek cures and you WILL find them.

The information I tell you proves itself 100% of the time to all those who use the information; who DO what the information tells you to do. I don't need people to pay attention to ME. You need YOU to pay attention to what I am sharing with you and put it to work for you. It works 100% of the time no matter how you get this information.

What I have noticed is that cures are also rare in books. Cures are not a part of our lives in the United States because doctors cure no one. But how could doctors cure anyone since cures are not taught in medical schools! We only get the things doctors are taught in medical schools. And the only thing doctors are good for when it comes to cures, is lab tests, diagnosis and for prescribing prescription drugs.

These are the only reasons I tell anyone to have anything to do with any doctors. Seeing a doctor WHILE you are curing yourself also keeps you from being so afraid. You would feel a whole lot better if doctors would be real doctors and just cure you. But since none of them will, you are all alone when you are curing yourself!

And although I am seeing more and more people learning exactly what I am teaching and used to cure myself of 11 chronic diseases, people like me are still not very common. This is how pathetic we have become as people and a nation. We no longer care about our health or lives, and use little cliches to pretend to justify the willful ignorance and contempt that made the people of this nation this way.

Poisoning ourselves to death is accepted because "we all gotta die sometime". And hey "nobody is gonna tell ME what I CAN and can NOT eat". But ask yourself this..... how's that working out for you? Gee, at least 150 Million Americans are permanently sick, while the rest of the nation is sick on a regular basis, until they are permanently sick the rest of their lives.

Your savage "American diet" and chlorinated fluoridated water did not work out for anyone! And the only ones these poisons didn't kill are the ones who were killed in accidents; 10% of this nation's people.

The United States is immersed in the worst plague of disease the planet has ever known. And even though it has been this way the past few decades, no one has sounded the alarm. No one has called this great plague a plague. And it's all because doctors never cure anyone.

And without any place to get cured, this monster plague of all time will continue to grow until every man, woman and child in the United States is permanently sick. And man's place on this Earth will continue to be made sick by corporations to maximize their profits, to then be used by doctors and the medical profession to also maximize their profits as their efforts continue killing 9 out of 10 Americans.

If at any time human life begins to matter, cures will solve the plague of chronic disease brought about by the willful incompetence and unbridled greed of doctors. This is easy to understand when you remember that about 85% of this country relied on healers until doctors and drug corporations began patenting their first drugs in 1939.

That brought the end of cures. And our nation's #1 natural medicine was made illegal, to force all Americans to get deadly chemical "medicines" that doctors and drug corporations make money off of, or suffer, or go to prison.

These fascists have fought their Treasonous war against The People, in the name of drugs, and filled our prisons to overflowing with pot smokers and dealers. This has just added to the suffering inflicted on The People. And the main ones who attack cures are those who profess to be christians.

It's bad enough that christians oppose cures. But when you remember they are suppose to be following the most well-known healer in the history of the planet, it becomes highly offensive to all decent people.

The thing Christ Jesus spent most of His time doing was curing the sick! He never "treated" the sick or told anyone "there is no cure". So you are either the devil himself OR you are willfully ignorant of that very bible you claim to believe! ALL those who do not hate Christ Jesus are in favor of cures, whether people are cured by believers laying their hands on the sick, or driving demons out of people, or if Nature cures them.

But to claim there are no cures, not even when they are proven and are Laws of Physics, is to point yourself out as not even being human. I make a point to refrain from talking about God, the bible or Spiritual things because I would never want anyone to think they have to know God to be cured. Any human can use these Laws of Physics to cure themselves Naturally.

The christian nonsense about claiming they dragged God into Hell and got God to "guide the hand of the surgeon" is vulgar. There is no claim in the bible that God ever guided the hand of any surgeon or even told you that butchery of your body was of any value! Surgeries make doctors big money. They are rarely of any value to your health unless you have been injured.

Doctors cut out cancer, tumors, cysts and other things because they REFUSE to cure you or even think about curing you. You have surgery to have a pacemaker put in because your doctor can't make any money off you taking Magnesium to insure proper rhythms. You have surgery to remove bladder stones, kidney stones and bone spurs because your doctors refused to cure you with Magnesium, Vitamin C and baking soda water.

So no use telling me your surgery did you any good! The people I know and have talked with have only suffered for months and years as a result of the high priced surgeries doctors assured them would help. But IF it helped, then why are they having the same surgery again!?! And why do people have to have one surgery after another, when your doctor said ONE surgery would solve your problem!?! I don't want you to suffer with one more surgery!

That's because the only possibility of me making any money off you is if you buy one of my books, or if you pay us at Cures R Us to provide you with as much assistance as you need until your body is restored to health and is rid of all disease. I could make a whole lot more money if I'd write one book for each step you must take to cure yourself! One book to tell you to take Magnesium. One to tell you to drink baking soda water. Another just to tell you to take Vitamin C. And a dozen others just to tell you what I have told you in this one book.

After all, when the only thing you care about is money, you make sure you get that first, then get some more. Your health and life do not matter to any doctor. If it did, they would cure you. It's just that simple. And restoring your body to health can be pretty simple, as long as you don't have doctors making it complicated.

When people contact me on Facebook to ask for my help and advice, most give me long explanations about all the disease names and other things their doctors told them. Only tid bits of what they tell me is of any value in getting them cured. This is because your diseases are the problem and not a part of the solution. So you must focus on your healing, not your diseases.

Thinking about the diseases you have only scares you. And thinking how the doctors said there's no cure and set a time frame from your death, just makes you that much more frightened. But in reality, the thing to be scared of is doctors and everything they do! But instead, people are afraid of Natural things, mostly because of the deliberate deceit of doctors.

The medical profession played a broken record to me about Natural things. My first Nephrologist confessed to having never learned medicine, when he stated that he had never learned about herbs, which are Natural medicines. That stunned me at the time. But throwing me out of the clinic he worked at, Clopton Clinic, topped that.

After I asked if there was an alternative to taking another drug to deal with the loss of Calcium another drug had caused, I soon got certified letters from both of my doctors at Clopton Clinic stating they would no longer be my doctors. What had really happened was that once they saw my blood tests confirmed that I was doing what THEY said could never happen, they threw me out of their clinic. They weren't interested in knowing how I did what I did.

Their official explanation said it was due to "non-compliance and general resistance to my recommendations for your care". Problem is, I did everything they told me to do. I was eager for their help and did everything they said to do because I thought they were going to cure me. Resisting was because I wanted to be cured not treated. Non-compliance was because I asked for an alternative to taking another drug for what a drug was causing.

They even put on my medical records that I didn't believe I had kidney disease and that I thought I was going to cure myself. Problem there is that I never thought for a second that I was going to cure myself. I didn't even think I had cured myself until about 3 years after I actually did! On top of that, it was doctors who I thought were going to cure me. At the time I thought that's what doctors did and was unaware that doctors refuse to cure anyone.

So saying I thought I was going to cure myself of a disease I didn't believe I had, just made me look crazy for sure. They stated on my medical records that I didn't think I had chronic kidney disease. It was because when they asked me "Do you think you have kidney disease?", I hesitated and looked at them funny and slowly said "That's what the doctors say."

I thought it was real odd to be asking such a question, much less going out of their way to lie about what I said. My medical records do NOT say I thought doctors would cure me OR that since doctors diagnosed me with chronic kidney disease, that I did indeed have chronic kidney disease. Why would my opinion about diagnosis of disease even matter?

So don't go pissing your doctor off by talking about something he knows nothing about and has never done and never WILL do....... curing someone! Go to doctors for the things they actually DO and don't allow yourself to waste your valuable time being angry at doctors for refusing to cure anyone.

It's the things you DO for yourself that get you cured, not the things or anything you stand against or oppose. So being angry at corporations and the medical profession for their behavior, is of no value in attaining your goal of freedom from all disease. Although I must admit that if we had a government in this country, we would not be devoid of all cures.

But it is each person who must learn to take care of their own body. You have to eat real food. And that means you have to learn what food is and where it comes from. The more you learn this, the more you learn that most of what you are eating and drinking originates in the laboratories of the food and drink corporations that make all these products.

I can make anyone sick in a few years just by telling them what to eat and drink. You need white flour, white sugar, high fructose corn syrup and red meat to insure chronic disease occurs. To make chronic disease occur even quicker I need to drink, cook and shower in unfiltered chlorinated fluoridated water. And I'll double up on the high fructose corn syrup by drinking some store bought fruit juice and soda pops.

But most Americans eat and drink like this and never think it's any big deal. Even when I had an excellent diet, within 5 years of drinking Ocean Spray juices, sodas, Gatorade and sugar sweetened tea every day, I had blown out my kidneys and was sitting on death's doorstep.

So how did I get from death's doorstep with dialysis my only choice besides death, to curing myself of 11 diseases doctors say there is no cure for? I wish the answer to that was that I sought a cure and found a cure. But that is not what I did. Sure I went to the doctor for a cure. But all they said was that there is no cure. And that is what every doctor told me.

So all I did was try whatever I could think of that might help me add some time onto my life, beyond the dialysis or death doctors gave me by 2008 or 9. In pursuit of that, I talked to a nurse that was in care of my mother when she passed away at age 85. It was the month after I was diagnosed with chronic kidney disease in October 2006.

As I was talking to the nurse about my mother, I told her how I had just been diagnosed with chronic kidney disease. She, Pat, said her husband had it too and was using ginger packs to soak the poisons out of his kidneys, to try and avoid dialysis. I got all excited and got every detail from her so I could start doing the same thing. But as I was looking for the ginger roots to begin, I started thinking "What if I never put the poisons IN my body. I wouldn't have to do anything to get them OUT of my body."

And for whatever reason, I became obsessed with keeping poisons OUT of my body. But I was at a loss as to where these poisons were coming from that I had to now keep out of my body. I had drank the Ocean Spray juices as an aid to my health. I drank the Gatorade to get all those "electrolytes". I drank the sodas because no one said not to or that they were bad for you, unless you want to lose weight.

And those 2 cups of white granulated sugar to sweeten a gallon of tea couldn't hurt me. So where are these poisons I need to keep out of my body? The mystery soon began to be solved when I drank some good ole Grape juice concentrate. I got it because I wanted a concentration of grape juice and was pretty sure that the concentrated Grape juice was healthy. So I started drinking it along with my Ocean Spray juices.

Yes, that's what I did. I kept right on drinking the most toxic thing I had been drinking the past few years, Ocean Spray Cranberry juice! But when I drank that Grape juice I noticed how that tense feeling I was working so hard to avoid, was as bad as it ever gets. The next time I drank the Grape juice I felt the same way. So I read the label again.

But I didn't know how it could be so toxic until I searched for the official FDA definition and saw that you could pack concentrate with all the sugar and high fructose corn syrup you choose, and toss in a small amount of fruit juice and sell it as "concentrate".

So that was the end of drinking any concentrated fruit juices. But I began to see what was causing that heightened tension. Every time I got that feeling was after drinking something with high fructose corn syrup in it. If something had white granulated sugar in it, the tension would be a bit heightened, but not as bad as high fructose corn syrup was.

I began avoiding high fructose corn syrup in lots of products. But I soon found that it was in almost all products. That's when the grocery store got real tiny. And my efforts to keep poisons OUT of my body suddenly turned in to the end of eating much of anything, or drinking anything besides water.

I hadn't eaten white flour since the very early 1980s. I know it is a drug, same as white granulated sugar is a drug. I didn't know anything about high fructose corn syrup. The facts later proved that it was high fructose corn syrup that had sent my blood pressure out of control and blown out my kidneys. But avoiding it wasn't the only thing I started doing.

I stopped cooking in the microwave, got organic soaps and shampoos, quit frying food in Teflon skillets, got a water filter and shower filter, and switched from whole milk to 2% milk. I also stopped drinking soda pops, Gatorade and sugar sweetened tea.

I had begun to search the INTERNET for curing kidney disease, avoiding dialysis and a few other similar terms. I never could find anything except for one book by Dr. Mackenzie Walser, whose book had "avoid dialysis" in the title. Then about a year later I found Dr. David Moskowitz, who had already given his clinically proven treatment to keep over 1000 US Veterans off of dialysis for up to 11 years.

But his bosses at the VA hospital had all these Veterans taken off Dr. Moskowitz's treatment. And as they slowly began to get worse and die, he left the VA and set out on his own and created GenoMed, Inc. And although he submitted all the information to the NIH to share with every doctor in the nation, the NIH later claimed they hadn't even heard of his work.

So our dear Veterans suffered and died needlessly because they are worth far more on dialysis for years, instead of this nation placing any value on their lives. Doing this to Veterans is the pinnacle of proof of how the entire medical profession places almost no value on your health or life. Their every decision is about what will make THEM the most money.

It was very humiliating for me when I was realizing these facts. But I got in touch with Dr. Moskowitz and got started on his drug treatment. It was a high dose of a common medication that is used to help control your blood pressure. When it is used in high doses, it inhibits the gene that is causing your kidney disease.

So I stayed on this drug treatment for 3 or 4 years while I worked on avoiding all the poisons I could. I began avoiding poisons in December of 2006. It was May 2008 when doctors threw me out of their clinic after having the proof that I was doing what they had never done, and what they said could NOT be done. I had reversed my kidney disease. But stupid me never heard anyone say there is a cure for kidney disease. So even though I was well on my way to being cured, I was oblivious to that fact.

I knew it was possible because I had ended my 4th bladder stone attack in 1996 with 2 Magnesium oxide vitamins and have not had another bladder stone attack to this day. That's 1996 to 2014. I call that a cure!

But even though I focused on my Creatinine and BUN, as they went lower and lower, I lost sight of what else was going on in my body. I did so just about all of 2009 and 2010. Then I started thinking about all the diseases I no longer had, and realized how much my health had improved. And to be quite honest, I hadn't drank any baking soda water during those years.

I learned about baking soda in 2012. I knew so little about it until then. I think about how much quicker I would have cured myself if I had just heard from anyone about drinking baking soda water! It was just like no one ever saying "Watch what you DRINK"! And that almost killed me. It's so easy to save people's lives and cure them. But we just don't do that because when it comes to disease, only what doctors say matters. And that has got to change if you ever want to be cured of any disease.

All cures are for your Natural body come from Nature. And all the things you need to restore your body to health are Natural. The chemicals you get from doctors are removed by your body completely; whereas all the Natural things are used by your body and become a part of your body. Only the excesses are removed by your body.

This is what I learned during those years I was trying to add some time to my life. I never thought about curing myself. So that caused me to cure myself of every disease I had, THEN look back and realize that is what I had done. I had my kidney disease in reverse. I only had slightly elevated BUN and Creatinine. So what else mattered?

Uh, I'll tell you what FINALLY mattered! The fact that I had not had any arthritis in 4 years (in 2010). And no headaches or heartburn in that time either. No intestinal bleeding. No bleeding gums. No more enlarged heart. No more being on the verge of Diabetes. I also cured myself of dandruff! I had not had any of these for the past 4 years, even though heartburn had been a daily thing. Same with bleeding gums and bleeding intestines. I had these the past 25 years, along with arthritis and headaches 3 or 4 days a week.

In 2006, my heart had become enlarged from excessively high blood pressure for an extended period of time. And I was on the verge of Diabetes since 2006 also. I also had gout once a year for the past ten years. I had it more often the last 3 or 4 years of my gout attacks.

I got rid of ALL of that in just about a year. But I didn't face up to what I had done until I had sustained that improvement for 3 years.

So I went back and thought about all that I had been doing, and started sorting out the things that helped, from the things that did not help. I also had to figure out just how they had helped and how valuable that help was.

That is when I started writing my first book, Self-Care HealthCare Guide. I wanted everyone to know what I had done, so that they could do the same for themselves and those around them. But the book didn't hardly sell at all. So I wrote a book about another subject and it sold OK. I was beginning to think it would be impossible to ever get this information to the Public.

I came up with the idea of spelling out what I had done to lead me to write that first book; which was that I had avoided dialysis. I also knew that I had cured myself of kidney disease. So that was the title of the book – How to Avoid Dialysis and Cure Kidney Disease. The title was to target a specific group of individuals that I was just a part of - people with kidney disease.

In that book is 3 chapters titled Poisons In Your Food, Drinks and Water. Those 3 chapters are in all 4 of my previous books on cures because they tell you the core of the cure for all diseases. It's those chapters that teach you how to clean up your food, drinks and water, which are the sources for the bulk of the poisons causing all disease.

Correcting your major diet deficiencies and learning how to avoid most poisons in your food, drinks and water, will almost insure your health will improve. And your health should continue to improve until all your diseases have faded away and are no longer any problem to you.

But if you make a habit of neglecting your body's needs and poison it again, you are going to get the SAME results you got before – headaches and heartburn, leading to worse diseases. Like I said earlier, I know how to make you sick. It's what led me to learn what cures all diseases.

I have no intention of ever asking the medical profession to change for the better. That hasn't happened because it's never going to happen. I believe the beginning of the problem is that you learn to trust doctors as though they are gods whose words are always true. And in doing so, doctors own you like a piece of meat on puppet strings and use you to maximize their income, but never attempt to cure you. And who is doing this? Yes, YOU are!

I'm not the only person who knows how to cure anyone of any disease. It use to be common for family members to know how to cure their loved ones. That's what we did as a nation before the first chemical drug was patented and the government locked down their monopoly with their fascist drug war. And almost overnight our nation's #1 medicine became illegal. Those who have not heeded this violently enforced drug monopoly, now fill our prisons to overflowing. All this in spite of monopolies being blatantly illegal.

The government knew that Cannabis oil cures cancer as early as 1974. But since this was irrelevant to Nixon's drug war, he buried the cure and set out to create propaganda to get his drug war going. Most of us know about the CIA getting caught smuggling in tons of Cocaine. They were trying to fool the Public into believing there was a need for this drug war of Nixon's.

Nixon chose instead to fabricate a report that would make it seem that smoking marijuana was at least as bad for you as cigarettes, and probably worse. And it worked, as this moron nation was blind to the fact of what was really going on. The whole nation let these government criminals not only ban our nation's #1 medicine, but let them make it illegal. And under the guise of battling the evil weed, our nation's #1 medicine has been the focus of their Nazi drug war against The People of the United States.

I don't want you to be overwhelmed by the history of this nation's stance against Natural medicine over the past 75 years. But I do want you to know these facts for a number of reasons.

I want you to know about the mere 75 years it has taken the efforts of a few Trillion dollars and your Police departments battling against The People, to enforce these drug corporation monopolies on everyone. I also want you to know how Truth can set you free of the entirety of everything they have done to eliminate Natural medicine and cures for The People. THEY are in a war against us. I am not in a war against them. I am active sharing the healing information of Natural Science that cures the Individual.

It's all science that doctors know and could tell you, but never do. But the reason we go to the doctor is to get cured. So I know it's insane to keep going to doctors for cures, when doctors cure no one! So even though doctors' behavior is a contradiction to their own title, you have to have a cure or remain sick. So don't let doctors' intolerance of cures affect you.

Get on with restoring your entire body to health as told in this book. And enjoy watching disease fade from your body. It's what you should have been doing all along. But since schools are for controlling children instead of teaching children, you aren't taught how to care for your own body. But then again, even the Constitution and Bill of Rights aren't taught in school!

Our schools COULD be useful, but all they do is focus on controlling others. And do so while they whine and complain about all the bullying and violence that trying to control others brings them. It's this obsession with controlling children that doesn't care about all the disease-causing garbage that make up school lunches.

I just saw an article in our local paper where they were saying how they were doing something about sodium, and had a picture of a kid and his lunch tray with a big carton of high fructose corn syrup saturated chocolate milk. But they didn't see that as a problem! Talk about focusing on a mole hill and ignoring the mountain! You can't get real food in schools because your school board members are in bed with the companies that sell the poisons!

Knowledge is Power. And the only Power I have for you is to empower you with the Truth and let the Truth set you free of all deceit; including all disease. The battle is not with corporations or doctors. The battle is inside YOU. The battle of YOU getting changed for the better by the Truth, self-evident facts.

Every one of you have gone to the doctor but never gotten cured. All I had to do was remind you of this self-evident fact we all know to be true. The most common attack against me and this information is to proclaim that I am a liar because there is no cure! Learn to cure yourself WHILE the medical profession continues shouting their incompetence that THEY cure no one. With THEM there are no cures, no possibility of you being cured.

I wanted you to know how I discovered this cure for all disease. I bought into their lies about there being no cures. I didn't even believe the facts I had lived for 3 or 4 years. I never even tried to cure myself of anything after I was diagnosed with kidney disease. I do not want that to happen to you.

I want you to know from the beginning that you are about to rid your body of all disease. It all depends on you changing. You change by learning facts to empower you and bring about that change.

Anyone has the Right to drink baking soda water to cure themselves. But why aren't most of us doing it! It's because doctors won't tell you to drink baking soda water. Yes they give it to all radiation patients to keep from killing all of them. Yes, doctors give it to almost all chemotherapy patients. Yes, doctors give it to dialysis patients. But they never tell their patients.

How would you feel if you realized that you were given baking soda water just so you stay alive to make doctors MORE money for more chemotherapy! It doesn't matter how you feel about it! It's what they do. You can't sue doctors for doing what all doctors do. Their State Medical Boards back them up on all use of medical procedures and excessive drugs.

So it's all up to YOU to cure yourself.

At first, knowing that made me feel kind of helpless and alone. I am always so thankful that I don't suffer from any of those 11 diseases I cured myself of. Just to still be alive is pretty amazing to me and my wife, after all I have been through since 2006. But to still be alive without a transplant or dialysis. And living without any disease at all in the past 6-7 years, is beyond amazing.

I don't think I am done writing books about cures; although I will be talking about how to have and maintain a healthy and disease-free body. Being buried in diseases and disease talk is just not necessary in my opinion.

What is important is that you know how to take care of your body. That means, it has to be a way of Life to make sure your body has all the nutrients it requires to be healthy. You also have to avoid poisons, since they are the cause of all disease. You have to have pure water, H2O; not H20 plus chlorine+fluoride. And you have to reverse the acidity of your body by drinking baking soda water until your body is free of all disease.

There have been people that have asked me for a cure for a certain disease, then asked me for a cure for another disease. I have given them the same cure for both of those diseases. That's because what I have been teaching you is the cure for all disease.

It's not that the "cure" is the same. It's that you restore your body to health the same way regardless of what disease or diseases you have. I have shown you how Magnesium, Vitamin C and Omega-3 cure quite a few diseases. And I have yet to find anyone who does not have these diet deficiencies. So until you give your body the things it needs, avoiding poisons is not going to rid your body of all diseases.

It's not poisons that cause improper heart rhythms. It's caused by a Magnesium deficiency. And although it is the fourth most plentiful nutrient in your body, you can't get enough Magnesium without taking vitamins. Same is true about Vitamin C. And you can't get enough Omega-3 unless you eat fish regularly. These deficiencies weaken your body and make it much easier for you to get sick.

So, this is where we always begin to rid your body of all disease. Add the baking soda water and filtered water and you have the foundation for every cure. But if you were taking care of your body in the first place, there would be no diseases and no need to cure any diseases. It's really all about giving your body what it needs and not bombarding it with lots of poisons.

It's the total number of poisons you put into your body that makes you sick. Your body is able to remove a large amount of poisons. But since our entire food, drinks and water supplies are saturated with poisons, these huge amounts of poisons have made the entire nation sick. And half the nation is permanently sick with "chronic" diseases. Most have more than one!

We are a vulgar nation that has sacrificed all the lives of The People of the United States, to be used by doctors and the medical profession to make as much money off The People as they can. They can't cure anyone because of all the money doctors would lose from YOUR healing!

I see no chance for anyone who trusts doctors. You really don't need a medical degree to cure all disease. You need reality; which is something that doesn't exist in the medical profession. Reality has no place in politics or religion either. And it's through religion and politics that this plague of chronic diseases have spread throughout the land and consumed the lives of us all.

It is up to The People if they ever choose to crawl out of the gutter and start caring for one another. No use to tell me you care about anyone when you won't even tell them there is a cure for all disease.

IF this nation is to ever crawl out of Hell, it has to begin with the health and well-being of The People. When christians should be working miracles to cure the sick, they are the most vicious opponents of cures. This is because Christ Jesus is the most well-known healer of the sick the planet has ever known. And since christians hate everything Christ Jesus did, they are totally intolerant of cures. Most doctors are christians. And doctors cure no one; not even if they claim to follow the most famous healer of all time!

This complete perversion by doctors is what keeps everybody from ever being cured of any disease. You think that if there was a cure for a disease that doctors would use that cure and cure you. But that is not true. The truth is that if doctors were more than doctors in name only, they WOULD cure most of their patients.

But since their perversion is total, your only hope for a cure is Nature. And once you realize that, it's between you and science.

I didn't know that doctors refuse to cure anyone until I went to them for a cure. That is when I experienced the fact that doctors have no cures. It's a very tough thing to endure when that means you will be dead real soon! But no matter how many millions of us go to doctors to be cured, not one doctor in the United States has cared about his patients over their unbridled greed.

There is no excuse for The People to continue without cures. And there is no excuse for any American to tolerate this fascist "drug war" that exists only to enforce drug corporations' illegal monopolies; and to use their drug war as the habitual excuse for violating the rights of millions of Americans each year.

I see no chance of the United States ever changing for the better. But you can make the choice to NOT be their victims. Use the information in this book to restore your body to health and thus rid it of all disease.

And deal with your food addictions. Do not continue to allow murderous corporations to kill you by saturating their products with deadly poisons and highly addictive drugs. You do not have to eat or drink their products.

You have a choice, as long as doctors are not your gods and you don't trust the FDA's claim that all these deadly poisons and highly addictive drugs are safe. It's sad to me that anyone has to tell you that poisons, chemicals, are not safe! You told yourself that if they weren't safe that the FDA would not allow it in any products.

But it's this big lie that has made the entire country sick, with half of the people permanently sick because doctors refuse to cure anyone.

Doctors could cure you. The problem is that curing you is not a money maker. It just helps The People. But when it comes to emergencies, the US has the best doctors in the world. So do yourselves a favor and know what value doctors really are. But when it comes to curing sickness, it's all up to you and science working together.

You have the knowledge to cure yourself of any and all disease. I hope you put it to work for you and your family.

You either listen to me, OR you stay sick and die many years before your time. Without the knowledge I have shared with you in this book, you have no chance of ever being well! It will take all of you to change that.

I can never have any sympathy for those who do not listen, because I can do nothing about anyone's freedom to make their own choices.

But before you reject The Cure For All Disease, remember that the only other choice you have is to stay sick the rest of your life.

No matter how much money you have, no one has ever bought a cure from doctors. No amount of money gets you a cure from doctors. But Nature and its Laws of Physics have been healing most people for several thousand years at least. That only changed since 1939.

So what's your choice going to be.....? cures of natures OR doctors and no chance of ever being cured?

Cures R Us – I have started a new company to help spread cures to all those who want to be cured. Cures R Us gives you the individual one-on-one help that most people want. We hope to open local offices soon and go out to people's homes and evaluate their food, drinks and water supplies, to teach you what is making you sick or WILL make you sick.

I am still working on the foundation for this one-of-a-kind business. This nation is devoid of cures. So a business to cure people has not existed in this nation since doctors abandoned all cures over the past 75 years.

There is no place for cures in this nation. Cures R Us has made a place for cures and hopes to bring cures into YOUR lives and the lives of those around you. Cures have to become a way of Life until this massive plague of chronic disease is wiped out by cures.

And with cures, comes the end of the medical profession as we know it. This is why they are more actively deceitful than ever. They want money, and cures won't ever satisfy the unbridled greed that rules all doctors.

I have accomplished what all doctors in this country combined have never done, cure chronic diseases. I have had the choice all along to believe this is because I am a much superior person than all doctors combined, OR that all doctors are greedy and perversely corrupt!

I certainly am superior to all doctors when it comes to cures and healing people. But I know I am not superior to all of you! I know of too many people that have cured themselves of chronic diseases much faster than I did.

These people are humble and speak highly of me and praise me with great praises for what I have taught them. But it is me that has even higher praise for THEM! They listened to ME. I listened to no one. I was all alone with no hope. I not only gave them hope, I gave them the knowledge that cured them. And now they tell everyone they can.

They are joyous about the end of their diseases. That joy is increased by the fact they didn't pay thousands or go bankrupt to be cured. And they are all joyous that they found cures for all the diseases that doctors have no cures for! For all of us, we have come out of the darkness and into the light concerning cures.

And it is for that goal that this book was written for YOU!

A cure is the ONLY thing that saves you from sickness and an early Death!

Spread the word – There is a cure for all disease.
And that cure cures ALL disease.

DISCLAIMER

There is nothing in this book that could be considered a violation of anyone's rights, or be construed as defamation, libel or illegal in any way, shape or form. All the objections to this book will come from doctors, nurses and their medical communities.

Anything that interferes with the unbridled greed of doctors, the medical profession, food and drink corporations or any corporation, is opposed and attacked. And this is the habitual behavior and treatment I have gotten from them. No doctor or nurse has ever shown any interest in curing anyone.

They insist that because THEY cure no one, that there are no cures at all. That lie is their basis for claiming I never cured myself, and/or that I never had any of the 11 diseases I cured myself of, or other baseless claims.

Fact is, that the medical profession are the ones who abandoned all cures and all natural, real, medicines over the past 75 years. And it is these facts that I have shared in this book.

It's doctors who are responsible for refusing to cure anyone anymore. I merely observed this fact and shared my experiences with doctors.

There is no attempt or intention by me to incite anyone to action against doctors, food and drink corporations or anyone or anything! I have made it clear that the only beneficial thing to do is avoid the products which corporations saturate with chemical poisons and highly addictive drugs. Avoid going to doctors expecting to ever be cured. And avoid all the other products made by corporations that are saturated with poisons.

My book is about empowering YOU, not leading you against all these doctors and corporations!

And the Right of The People to share knowledge that makes life better for all those who embrace it, can not be subjugated beneath a tyrannical despotism that prevents The People from our pursuit of life, liberty and happiness. It is in that Spirit that this book is written.

All the information is proven science that has been around since time began; and used by man for many centuries. Any information other than that is written from my own personal experiences.

No material has been copied from anyone else or any copyrighted source of materials or information.

This book was written to guide people in doing the things that will improve their health and cure them, if they are willing to do the natural things it takes to do so. While there are some facts stated in here that are critical of some things, there is absolutely no intent to defame or misrepresent the facts about these persons, companies or others.

On the contrary, I intentionally left out the names of the companies saturating our food, drinks and water supplies. I did this so that no one would think that talking to these people or companies is of any real value. So, if anyone takes anything said in this book to mean to defame, misrepresent or anything of that nature, they are only stating their opinion of what is in this book, but not stating an opinion based on facts.

I am fully aware of how the people in the medical profession, generally and according to my own experiences, will attack and criticize anything that is not something they do and make money off of. I have no interest in their drama and choose to avoid it altogether.

I have never told anyone to stop going to the doctor. On the contrary, I tell them to cure themselves WHILE they still do what the doctors say for them to do. I'm not afraid of doctors. I just know not to look to doctors or the medical profession for cures.

No one should, in any way, take anything stated in this book as promoting or even suggesting any type of action toward any part of government, companies, doctors or the likes.

On the contrary, I suggest you stop buying products with the disease causing poisons pointed out in this book. And no one should be so twisted and perverted in their minds to claim that Individuals do not have the Right to protect ourselves from disease-causing poisons and all poisons.

This book places absolutely ZERO HOPE that food companies will ever make the choices to remove the poisons from their products. So, the only choice we have is to freely share the knowledge individuals need to avoid the poisons in food and drink products.

Just because doctors and the rest of the medical profession don't get to make money off the diseases I cure, prevent or never have, does not constitute any illegal or inappropriate act or acts.

www.ingramcontent.com/pod-product-compliance
Lightning Source LLC
Chambersburg PA
CBHW081849170526
45167CB00007B/2944